REIMAGINING REPRODUCTION

This book presents an ethnographic study on gestational surrogacy in India. It frames the ethnography of the surrogacy clinic in conversation with concerns raised in the arenas of law, policy, medical ethics, and global structural inequality about the ethics of transnational assisted reproductive technology (ART) practices. Engaging ethical discourses that both advocate for and trouble the subject of reproductive rights that remains of interest in feminist studies, the volume takes up the work of critical feminist, anthropological and science studies scholarship in India, the United States, and Europe concerned with reproductive technologies.

Based on fieldwork and archival sources, the volume will be of great interest to scholars and researchers of ethnography, gender, social and public policy, South Asian studies, and global public health, especially reproductive health.

Kalindi Vora is Professor of Ethnicity Race & Migration, Women's Gender and Sexuality Studies, History of Science and Medicine, and American Studies at Yale University. She is author of *Life Support: Biocapital and the New History of Outsourcing*, *Reimagining Reproduction: Essays on Surrogacy, Labor and Technologies of Human Reproduction*, and co- author of *Surrogate Humanity: Race, Robots, and the Politics of Technological Futures*. With the Precarity Lab, she is author of *Technoprecarious*.

REIMAGINING REPRODUCTION

Essays on Surrogacy, Labor, and Technologies of Human Reproduction

Kalindi Vora

Routledge
Taylor & Francis Group
LONDON AND NEW YORK

First published 2023
by Routledge
4 Park Square, Milton Park, Abingdon, Oxon OX14 4RN

and by Routledge
605 Third Avenue, New York, NY 10158

Routledge is an imprint of the Taylor & Francis Group, an informa business

British Library Cataloguing-in-Publication Data
A catalogue record for this book is available from the British Library

ISBN: 978-1-032-37907-4 (hbk)
ISBN: 978-1-032-40498-1 (pbk)
ISBN: 978-1-003-35336-2 (ebk)

DOI: 10.4324/9781003353362

Typeset in Sabon
by Apex CoVantage, LLC

In memoriam: Christine Ann (Stromberg) Snell

CONTENTS

ACKNOWLEDGMENTS

In Ahmedabad, my thanks to Ramesh Bhakta for offering me generous support after we were introduced by our shared friend Matt Rahaim; and to Nishant Shah, in Ahmedabad and everywhere else, for animated conversation and hospitality. In Rajkot: Kirit, Kanak, and Nishad Vohra, my gratitude for always having an open door and welcoming me to be with family. In "northwestern India," to the necessarily anonymous surrogates, doctors, staff, and commissioning parents who shared their thoughts and stories with me, I feel ongoing gratitude and responsibility to share them accurately, and I hope I've done them justice.

Colleagues who've supported this work between 2008-2016 can be found across the world. My writing group at UC Berkeley in 2008-2009, including Neda Atanasoski, Kim Tallbear and Elly Teman, read and commented on some my first attempts at writing through this research. My first invitation to present this research was by the Barnard Feminist and Scholar conference titled, "Critical Conceptions: Technology, Justice, and the Global Reproductive Market," through Neferti Tadiar, whose invitation inspired the first piece I published out of this research in their journal *The Scholar & Feminist* Online, included here as chapter two. Also early in this research, Sheela Saravanan invited me to speak on a panel for the 2010 European Conference on Modern South Asian Studies that she organized titled, "Reproductive Tourism in India: Ethical and Legal Concerns." In 2011, Karen Sue Taussig and Klaus Hoeyer invited me to be a part of the Wenner-Gren symposium "The Anthropology of Potentiality," whose powerful week long workshop and ensuing special issue of *Current Anthropology* provoked another article included as chapter six in this collection. Also in 2011, Kay Warren and the Pembroke Center at Brown invited me to present at its annual symposium in with the theme *Global Relations: Kinship and Transnationalism,* where I benefitted from deep conversations and productive feedback. I also received tremendous benefit from invitations to present this work at the UC Berkeley Center for Race and Gender conference titled, Speculative Visions of Race, Technology, Science and

Survival in 2013, and at the symposium titled, "Habits of Living: Networked Affects, Glocal Effects" organized by Wendy Chun and Nishant Shah at Brown University in 2013. Marlene Jouan invited me to join the conference titled, Women's and Mothers' Labor: the Stakes of Surrogacy" at Grenoble Alpes University France in 2017, and Cressida Limon invited me to present at Eggs, Milk and Honey: Law and Global Biocommodities at Western Sydney University in 2018. Both of these events offered meaningful and productive conversations around the intersections of assisted reproduction, medical travel, law, and ethics across borders.

Many pieces in this collection have benefitted from the generous editorial feedback of colleagues who shepherded them through publication in special journal issues. Maria Puig della bella Casa solicited a piece for *Subjectivities*, included here as chapter three, and Melinda Cooper and Terry Woronov invited me to contribute to their special issue of South Atlantic Quarterly titled, "Labor's Contingency: New Spaces and Times of Work." That piece is include here as chapter four. My thanks also to Fouziehya Towghi for endurance lasting from the 2008 Society for Medical Anthropology conference panel we co-organized through the special issue of the journal *Ethnos* we edited and finally published in 2014, including the article I've included here as chapter seven. Damien W. Riggs and Donna McCormack my contribution to their special issue of *Somatechnics*, titled, "The Ethics of Biomedical Tourism," for which I wrote *Re-imagining Reproduction*, here as chapter five. Nina Lykke and Merete Lie solicited a contribution from me for their edited volume with Routledge titled, *Assisted Reproduction Across Borders: Feminist Perspectives on Normalizations, Disruptions, and Transmissions,* and Malathi Iyengar generously agreed to collaborate with me to write "Citizen, Subject, Property," which appears here as chapter eight. Brenna Bhandar asked me to contribute to the dossier she organized for *Radical Philosophy* with the goal of highlighting the forty years of materialist, Black, and women of color scholarship that has built a foundation of feminist theories of social reproduction, a history sometimes overlooked even among feminist scholars. Chapter nine, "After the Housewife," originally appeared in that dossier, and Brenn Bhandar's editorial feedback was indispensable. I also thank my colleagues in the department of Ethnic Studies at UC San Diego from 2009-2016, especially Yen Espiritu, Roshanak Kheshti, and Saiba Varma who offered comments on some of the pieces, and to those who taught some of these pieces to our students, including Jillian Hernandez, Sara Clarke Kaplan, Kirstie Dorr, Curtis Marez, Shelley Streeby, Daphne Taylor-Garcia and Wayne Yang.

For love and moral support during the decade I pursued this research: Neda Atanasoski, Amy Pavlakovich, Julie Murphy, Alex Vora, Christine Vora, Kavi Vora Camp, Nathan Camp, Naruna Vora Camp, and Nisheeth Vora.

1

INTRODUCTION

Mixing intimacy and business, but also bodies and technologies, commercial surrogacy arrangements are occurring worldwide amidst competing claims about the meaning of parenthood, the value of mothering and of the child, and the moral and ethical implications of reproductive technologies. Indian transnational surrogacy arrangements, at their height between 2008 and 2016 when the Indian government passed legislation disallowing transnational contracts, illustrate important issues for the future of transnational surrogacy. The crossing of cultural norms, government regulations, and legal structures established case law precedent and global expectations for what might occur to commissioning parents and surrogates. Since it caters to clients from wealthier nations, transnational Indian surrogacy arrangements require attention to the politics and economics of the global division of reproductive labor. For example, when a person from the United States or United Kingdom hires an Indian woman to carry a child by in vitro fertilization (IVF) commercially, on one level it is an exchange of services for payment. On another, the surrogate mother is doing work that enhances and actually reproduces the life of that person or family. For women working as surrogates, surrogacy also requires the re-conceptualization of their own bodies and their relationship to childbirth. As a result, she reconstitutes her relationship to her body and to the meaning of childbirth to effectively contributing to the enrichment and longevity of the US or UK economy and society. The Indian surrogacy market has also come to be understood as a lens and a metaphor for longer histories of racial capitalism's investment in capturing the reproductive power and potential of women's bodies.[1]

Surrogacy was legalized in India in 2002, and in 2004 a successful case of surrogacy in a small Indian fertility clinic grew quickly into an industry. The mother of a woman living in the United Kingdom desired a pregnancy but had uterine problems approached her local fertility clinic in India on behalf of her daughter and her daughter's Indian-origin husband. The directors of the clinic had been performing IVF for diasporic Indians, and agreed to try the surrogacy, which ended in the successful birth of a child for these UK citizens by an Indian citizen, the grandmother of the infant. The

DOI: 10.4324/9781003353362-1

care got transnational attention, and by 2008, India's national government needed to draft legislation to regulate the many small clinics springing up to arrange surrogacy with Indian women for international citizens who desired an infant sharing their genetic material. Transnational surrogacy arrangements between Indian surrogates and non-Indian commissioning parents were banned by the government at the end of 2015. Recently, "Social Reproductive Theory" or SRT was coined as a term to reference what seems like capitalism's new interest in the reproductive capacities of the human body,[2] though feminist materialists have been examining reproductive labor and producing theories about the role of reproduction and reproductive labor under capitalism since the 1970s. The essays about Indian transnational surrogacy herein engage 40 years of material feminist, Black feminist and women of color feminist materialist theories of how reproduction has always been at the center of capitalism's engines, if obscured by social and cultural devaluing of reproductive work and bodies. To those newly discovering the imbrication of social and material reproductivity in the history of racial capitalism, I hope these essays will expand and enrich that process, both in terms of regions and in terms of bodies of feminist theory.

Commercial surrogacy is out of the financial reach of most middle-class citizens in countries where it is legal. The medical process of surrogacy requires IVF, where a human egg is inseminated under a microscope by an embryologist, who then cultures the embryo until it is ready to be transplanted into the uterus of a woman, the gestational surrogate. She must undergo hormone therapy to prepare her uterus so that the embryo can attach, resulting in pregnancy. Intending parents may also need to buy or recruit gametes, human eggs, sperm, or both, in order to begin the process of surrogacy. Not only do these techniques and practices require access to money, technology, and medical specialists, but they also require commissioning parents to navigate legal risk and uncertainty as they redefine reproduction while moving across international borders and through distinct legal systems and understandings of citizenship.

Women enter commercial surrogacy contracts for a spectrum of reasons, impelled by a matrix of local and national social and economic factors. The possibility of becoming a surrogate as a form of paid service is often discovered through word-of-mouth when someone in a given community completes a pregnancy and delivery as surrogate. Women from that community may then begin to understand surrogacy as a way to establish economic security and self-recruit to approach surrogacy clinics. Women interested in working as surrogates, whom depending on the clinic may be day laborers from rural communities with a middle school- or high school-equivalent education or college educated women from more urban areas, are introduced to the process of surrogacy. Using IVF with an ovum from a donor or commissioning mother, the ensuing embryo is then transplanted to her uterus with the assistance of hormone injections that will allow the embryo to implant. Some clinics, including the clinic I worked with, also interview a potential surrogate's husband, and her contract requires his signed consent. The introduction to assisted reproduction is meant to help them both to understand that surrogacy does not involve their bodies sexually, and also to encourage them to emotionally distance themselves from the commissioning infant. As explained in Chapter 3, medical staff encourage surrogates to see themselves as gestation-providers whose only link to the fetus is the lending of their womb for its development until it is born.

After becoming surrogates, women often relocate to live in designated housing close to the clinic to ease their daily work load and its risks to the pregnancy, and to easily access prenatal care. As described in Chapter 3, women I spoke to felt the hardship of being away from their families and communities, but also the necessity of keeping this work for reasons of stigma. Despite seeing the work as morally defensible themselves, a number of women felt it would be impossible to gain the same understanding outside the clinic.

Most of the commissioning parents who come to India to hire surrogates are heterosexual couples in which the intended mother is unable to carry a fetus to term; in the clinic where I was based, this was a condition to be considered for a surrogacy arrangement. Some choose to arrange for surrogacy in India because commercial surrogacy is illegal in their home countries. Commissioning parents from abroad described choosing an Indian surrogacy clinic over those in their home countries or other transnational surrogacy destinations for economic, medical, legal, and psychological reasons. Both IVF and contracting with a surrogate were described as significantly less costly in India when compared to their home countries. In some countries like the United States, the legal precedent of surrogates having successfully sued for custody rights to the child they carried made commissioning parents feel legally more secure contracting a surrogate in India. For similar reasons, other commissioning parents wanted to raise their children with the significant social and geographical distance between their home countries and that of their surrogate. These push and pull factors for commissioning parents, as well as for women entering surrogacy contracts, are detailed in Chapter 3, and discussed further in later chapters.

The work of gestation and nurture becomes visible in commercial surrogacy in a way that it may not be within a nuclear family and household. Once commodified, this work of care also becomes subject to the alienation of capitalist relations. What are the social and economic implications of alienation in the work of mothering in surrogacy? Does the opportunity to sell gestation and nurture for a low price globally lower the value of non-commercial mothering? Assisted reproductive technologies allow women to sell the service of gestating a fetus, but legal precedent regarding custody, and medical emphasis on genetic connection, means that surrogates maintain little or no claim to the product of that labor: the child itself. In the context of transnational Indian surrogacy, this situation is more extreme because of the physical and cultural distance between intended parents and surrogates.

This volume is composed of a series of ethnographic essays from my research on gestation surrogacy between 2008 and 2016. Until now, this research, which represents one of the small number of original ethnographic studies of transnational surrogacy in India, was published exclusively in articles, which has made them difficult to access as a complete study. It frames the ethnography of the surrogacy clinic in conversation with concerns raised in the arenas of law, policy, medical ethics, and global structural inequality about the ethics of transnational ART practices. Engaging ethical discourses that both advocate for and trouble the subject of reproductive rights that remains of interest in feminist studies, the volume takes up the work of several mainstream and feminist advocacy and science policy watchdog groups in India, the United States, and Europe concerned with reproductive technologies.

In October 2020, at the time of writing, an article-length study was published offering a new framework of Dalit feminist frameworks for reproductive justice, a valuable and necessary approach to surrogacy and egg donation in India. It addresses the gap in attention to caste in favor of the focus on class and economic status among existing ethnography and interviews on the topics.[3] Caste appears in the essays in this volume as a sociological marker used by participants and interviewees, usually not explicitly, but implicitly through reference to phenotypical traits, eye-color, skin-tone, or vegetarian diet. The ethnography was conducted exclusively with participants in transnational surrogacy arrangements, and caste as an identity is marked more explicitly in ethnographies including arrangements between Indian commissioning parents and surrogates.[4] The contribution of a Dalit feminist lens on ART in India, based on the authors' interviews with Dalit feminists about egg donation and surrogacy in India, forward new frameworks for considering the structural role of caste in India's reproductive politics at large, even when the caste of individuals in a given ethnographic context may not assert itself as central. For example, within domestic Indian surrogacy arrangements, women and men with "caste capital" are protected from the economic and social vulnerability that most often necessitates the selling of eggs and the entry into surrogacy contracts. Gondouin et al. call this the "brahminization of surrogacy," in which new roles are created for lower caste women while confining them within the frame of "non-valuable breeders" for the embryos of "valuable" women.[5]

A Dalit feminist approach to reproductive justice, as advanced by Gondouin, Thapar-Bjorkert, and Mohan Rao in India's context, must work through caste abolition. Understandings of caste, as described in Ambedkar's writings, are grounded in caste endogamy. This makes the control of women's sexuality central to caste ideology.[6] Applying Dalit feminists frameworks means interrogating the privilege and discrimination embedded within the Ambedkarian notion of "Brahminical patriarchy," that is, a form of patriarchy unique to the subcontinent that is an organization of gendered hierarchy through a simultaneous set of discriminatory levels organizing society based on caste.[7] The framework of reproductive justice as a project of caste abolition in India, given the history of oppression and exploitation of women's sexuality and reproductivity through caste and gender as inseparable,[8] is an essential and overdue addition to the theorizing of transnational biocapital markets as they draw upon the reproductivity of Indian women. As Gondouin, Thapar-Bjorkert, and Mohan Rao rightly point out, analysis of surrogacy and egg donation must engage a theoretical framework that includes the history of caste oppression as inherent to gender and reproduction in the subcontinent given the history of casteist eugenicism, as well as more recent Hindu nationalist assertions of caste supremacy that construct oppressed castes as unfit to reproduce.[9]

In 2016, after my study concluded, the Indian Surrogacy (Regulation) Bill was passed to ban all commercial surrogacy in the country and the contracting of surrogacy arrangements between Indians and foreigners. Only altruistic surrogacy for married couples with documented infertility who worked with a close relative as their surrogate would be legal. Gondouin et al. describe this and the revised version of the bill passed in August 2019 as assigning Indian women's reproductive responsibilities to the nation, rather than as reproducers for the global bioeconomy. Banerjee and Kotiswaran pointed out that the 2019 Surrogacy Regulation bill fails to incorporate the recommendations of two reports representing 50 members of parliament, and does not address the related lack of updated regulations for assisted reproductive technologies (ARTs), meaning that the Bill "will be tied up in constitutional regulation for years."[10] This collection of essays relies on ethnographic narratives collected in 2008, and continuing analysis until 2016, and works with news and popular media, legal case law, and feminist science and technology studies perspectives to give readers a first-hand sense of the experience and motivations of doctors running surrogacy clinics, women who have been surrogates, and the people who travel to India to have children via Indian surrogacy. Each essay contains an independent methodology and argument, but together the essays situate the growth of commercial surrogacy in India within discussions of the economic and legal debates happening around surrogacy in India and in the home countries of commissioning parents. It is intended to inform researchers in transnational surrogacy and ARTs, and is also appropriate for undergraduate courses in international studies, women and gender studies, international relations, and any course teaching material on medical tourism and ethics, global health, and labor politics. Because the text is based on narratives, the main ideas about the transnational economy of care and labor at work in transnational surrogacy are meant to be accessible to readers who have no background in the topics of gender, labor, and reproduction.

***

Chapter 2, *Medicine, Markets, and the Pregnant Body*, outlines the process at the Manushi clinic, then looks at how commercial surrogacy in India relies on a western medical understanding of the body that constructs the uterus as surplus, and a genetics-based model of parentage that creates a connection between the intended parents and fetus, and a distance between the surrogate and the fetus. The essay then focused specifically on how the clinic portrays its surrogacy practice as a form of social work, emphasizing the ways that fees paid to surrogates through the clinic materially improve their lives rather than serving only as wages and profit to the clinic, and the ways that the understanding of the divine nature of the act of surrogacy provides another narrative of the meaning and value of commercial surrogacy outside of market logic.

Chapter 3, *The Commodification of Biological and Affective Labor*, looks at how reproductive technologies allow women to sell the service of gestating a fetus but maintain little or no claim to the product of that labor: the child itself. In the context of transnational Indian surrogacy, this situation is exacerbated by the physical and cultural distance between intended parents and surrogates. The productive nature of the care and nurturing provided through the unpaid work of mothering becomes more visible when viewed though the commodification of commercial surrogacy. Once commodified, this work of care also becomes subject to the alienation of capitalist relations, which invites us to investigate the social and economic implications of the work of mothering in surrogacy. This chapter argues that care and nurture in transnational Indian surrogacy invest human vital energy as a form of value directly into other human beings, through the biological and affective labor involved in surrogate work, thereby supporting the lives of those individuals, families, and societies that consume this energy.

Chapter 4, *Limits of "Labor": Accounting for Affect and the Biological in Transnational Surrogacy and Service Work*, looks at how affective and biological labor found in call center and surrogacy work index new forms of exploitation and accumulation within neoliberal globalization, while simultaneously rearticulating the history of a colonial division of labor. This chapter argues that tracking vital energy, rather than value, as the content of what is produced and transmitted between biological and affective producers and their consumers holds on to the human vitality that Marx describes as the content of value carried by the commodity, while also describing the content of these value-producing activities as greater than what can be described in terms of physical commodities and their value as represented through exchange. Feminist materialist scholarship and critiques of the racialized nature of domesticity and free labor advanced by feminists based on the Global South, Black feminists, and US women-of-color feminists provide the ground for continuing to scrutinize which kinds of exchange and subjectivity can even be represented by categories of labor.

Chapter 5, *Re-imagining Reproduction: Unsettling Metaphors in the History of Imperial Science and Commercial Surrogacy in India*, takes a feminist science and technology studies approach to examining the way that the pregnant body, the fetus, and the physician are figured in the ART clinic. Building on the work of historian of colonial medicine in India Gyan Prakash and David Arnold, it follows the coloniality of medicine into the present-day shift in medicine from a technique of caring for the body to one of producing bodies as the instruments of service work. In this context, the body of the surrogate is rendered available as part of an experimental economy of gestation as a service, provided by the surrogate as entrepreneur, all of which is enabled in part by the continuing relationship between medicine and the colonization of bodies in India.

Chapter 6, *Potential, Risk, and Return*, brings together ethnography and analysis of assisted reproductive technology (ART) legislation under consideration in the Indian parliament, this chapter examines how bodies become potentialized through a combination of technology and networks of social and economic inequality. In this process, the meaning that participants assign to bodies and social relationships mediated by bodies becomes destabilized in a way that allows some surrogates to imagine and work toward a connection to commissioning parents that will offer them long-term benefit. The politics that position the clinic to potentialize the bodies of surrogates—and as a result the relations between participants and their imagined outcomes—occur at a moment of global demand for ARTs. As such, they rely on differentiation of subjects culturally, geographically, and economically.

Chapter 7, *Experimental Sociality in the Indian Surrogacy Clinic*, marks experimental modes of sociality in the clinic as a contact zone between elite doctors, gestational surrogates, and transnational commissioning parents. It examines efforts to separate social relationships from reproductive bodies in its surrogacy arrangements as well as at novel social formations occurring both because of and despite these efforts. The clinic provides an opportunity to observe forms of sociality that emerge as experiments with modernities, with different relationships to the body and the social meaning of medicalized biological reproduction, and with understanding the role of the market and altruism in the practice of gestational surrogacy.

Chapter 8, *Citizen, Subject, Property* (co-authored with Malathi Iyenger), argue that when US commissioning parents contract Indian women as commercial gestational surrogates, they engage a structural history of the instrumentalization of the reproductive capacities of women who are marginalized by race, class, and the law for the benefit of subjects who are economically, legally, and socially more privileged. Putting analysis of the practice of US commissioning parents contracting commercial surrogacy in

India into conversation with theories of citizenship and the nation-state, focusing in particular on US citizenship and its racial underpinnings, we not only suggest lines of inquiry for the ongoing scholarly examination of transnational surrogacy, but also suggest that discourses of citizenship might be strategically deployed in the policy arena in order to pursue a greater measure of rights and benefits for gestational mothers.

Chapter 9, *Conclusion: After the Housewife*, discusses the political difficulties with approaching surrogacy only as a labor rights topic, particularly within the context of women of color feminist theory. Briefly tracing the history of feminist theories of reproductive labor and women of color feminist assertions of the need for understanding these subjects as providing more-than-labor in different ways, the chapter pushes us to think about the problems and potentials of commercial surrogacy with and beyond feminist theories of labor and social reproduction.

Notes

1 Federici 2004.
2 Bhattacharya 2017.
3 Authors cite Pande 2014; Rudrappa 2015; Vora 2015; Deomampo 2016. The Vora (2015) citation refers to my book about outsourcing, *Life Support*, and not any of the articles included in this volume.
4 See Pande 2014; Rudrappa 2015; SAMA 2012.
5 Corea 1985, 276, cited by Gondouin et al. 2020, 10.
6 Rege 1998, 165; Velayudhan 2018, cited Gondouin et al. 2020, 6.
7 Arya and Rathore 2020, 8, cited by Gondouin et al. 2020, 5.
8 Gondouin et al. 2020, 6.
9 Authors explain that within domestic Indian surrogacy arrangements, intended parents would ideally prefer a higher caste or Brahmin surrogate, with the expectation that they would produce "healthy and good-looking babies" (Dhar 2012, cited by Gondouin et al. (2020, 9–10)). Interviewees describe "Brahmin eggs" and "Brahmin sperm" versus the womb of the lower-caste woman, whose caste impurity, imagined through impure sexuality, makes her own eggs undesirable (Ibid.). Authors suggest "that these reproductive practices assist in building "caste capital," which confers benefits comparable to those accrued from social capital (Ibid.).
10 Sneha Banerjee and Prabha Kotiswaran. (2020). "Divine Labours, Devalued Work: The Continuing Saga of India's Surrogacy Regulation," *Indian Law Review*, DOI:10.1080/24730580.2020.1843317.

Works Cited

Arya, Sunaina and Aakash Singh Rathore. (2020). "Introduction," in *Dalit Feminist Theory: A Reader*. London: Routledge, pp. 173–182.

Banerjee, Sneha and Prabha Kotiswaran. (2020). "Divine Labours, Devalued Work: The Continuing Saga of India's Surrogacy Regulation," *Indian Law Review*. DOI: 10.1080/24730580.2020.18433.

Bhattacharya, Tithi. (2017). *Social Reproduction Theory: Remapping Class, Recentering Oppression*. London: Pluto Press.

Corea, Gena. (1985). *The Mother Machine: Reproductive Technologies from Artificial Insemination to Artificial Wombs*. New York: Harper & Row.

Deomampo, Daisy. (2016). *Transnational Reproduction: Race, Kinship and Commercial Surrogacy in India*. New York: New York University Press.

Dhar, Aarti. (2012). "Beautiful and Fair' Preferred Among Surrogate Mothers Too," *The Hindu*, October 25. www.thehindu.com/sci-tech/health/policy-and-issues/beautiful-and-fair-preferred-among-surrogate-motherstoo/article4028640.ece.

Federici, Sylvia. (2004). *Caliban and the Witch: Women, the Body and Primitive Accumulation*. New York: Autonomedia.

Gondouin, Joanna, Suruchi Thapar-Bjorkert and Mohan Rao. (2020). "Dalit Feminist Voices of Reproductive Rights and Reproductive Justice," *Economic and Political Weekly*, 6, October 3.

Murphy, Michelle. (2017). *The Economization of Life*. Durham and London: Duke University Press.

Pande, Amrita. (2014). *Wombs in Labour: Transnational Commercial Surrogacy in India*. New York: Colombia University Press.

Rege, Sharmila. (1998). "Dalit Women Talk Differently: A Critique of 'Difference' and Towards a Dalit Feminist Standpoint Position," *Economic & Political Weekly*, WS39–WS46, October 31.

Roberts, Dorothy E. (1996). "Race and the New Reproduction," *Hastings Law Journal*, 47(4): 935–949.

Rudrappa, Sharmila. (2015). *Discounted Life: The Price of Global Surrogacy in India*. New York and London: New York University Press.

SAMA. (2012). *Birthing a Market: A Study of Commercial Surrogacy*. New Delhi: SAMA-Resource Group for Women and Health.

Twine, France Winddance. (2011). *Outsourcing the Womb: Race, Class and Gestational Surrogacy in a Global Market*. New York and London: Routledge.

Velayudhan, Meera. (2018). "Linking Radical Traditions and the Contemporary Dalit Women's Movement: An Intergenerational Lens," *Feminist Review*, 119: 106–125.

Vora, Kalindi. (2015). *Life Support: Biocapital and the New History of Outsourced Labor*. Minneapolis and London: University of Minnesota Press.

Weinbaum, Alys Eve. (2019). *The Afterlife of Reproductive Slavery: Biocapitalism and Black Feminism's Philosophy of History*. Durham and London: Duke University Press.

2

MEDICINE, MARKETS, AND THE PREGNANT BODY

Indian Commercial Surrogacy and Reproductive Labor in a Transnational Frame

In early 2008, I observed and interviewed doctors, lab technicians, clinic staff, and commissioning parents who were in the process of having a child through a surrogate, and women working as surrogates at the Manushi fertility clinic in northern India.[1] In the tradition of medical anthropology, I approach the clinic as a contact zone where unique interactions and relationships occur, and these constitute the center of my study. In the tradition of both subaltern historiographies and feminist methodologies, I aim to point to possibilities in the subject positions of those from whom I learned during fieldwork without representing this knowledge as anything but a particular reading produced from my context as a scholar based in the United States.

At the time, transnational commercial surrogacy in India was a small but growing industry that had attracting media attention as part of a larger popular interest in surrogacy in the United States and elsewhere. The doctors at the clinic in northern India where I did fieldwork in early 2008 were aware of a handful of other clinics at that time in the Indian cities of Chennai, Mumbai, Hyderabad, and Ahmedabad. The path for this industry was paved by already-existing infrastructures of transportation and communication, discourses about outsourcing and the cheapness of Indian labor, and epistemologies of the body and kinship as they have been influenced by western science and medicine. These conditions of possibility are interwoven with the continued development of biotechnologies of human reproduction in ways that increase the choices of those with access to these technologies. For women implicated in new technologies through the biological materials or labor they provide, for example, through the roles of egg donor or gestational surrogate, advances in reproductive technologies can increase the range of income options while simultaneously compromising the desirability of these options. The enabling conditions for transnational surrogacy occur in a context of contested cultural domains, where multiple understandings of the significance and social meaning of reproductive technologies have to

DOI: 10.4324/9781003353362-2

vie for traction. By tracing some of these understandings, this article considers how transnational Indian surrogacy reflects aspects of the privatization and commodification of reproduction and reproductive labor.

Scholarship on assisted reproduction in India suggests that for the middle class elites who can afford them, assisted reproductive technologies can reduce the social stigma for otherwise childless married women and help provide old-age security for couples who have been unable to have children in other ways (Inhorn and Bharadwaj 2007). There is evidence that the reach of these technologies is expanding (Bharadwaj 2000), but the economic constraints on the women who become surrogate mothers means that women in their social and economic strata are not candidates for the potential benefit of these technologies themselves (Inhorn et al. 2008; Spar 2006), and it therefore serves as another example of "stratified reproduction" (Colen 1995).

This chapter outlines the surrogacy process at the Manushi clinic, and overviews common themes in the following essay-based chapters. It introduces how commercial surrogacy in India relies on a western medical understanding of the body that constructs the uterus as surplus, and a genetics-based model of parentage that creates a connection between the intended parents and fetus and a distance between the surrogate and the fetus. It opens up the question of what is the nature of surrogacy as paid work versus a noncommercial offering, a theme across the chapters, as well as in surrogacy scholarship at large. For example, the clinic portrays surrogacy as a form of social work, emphasizing the ways that fees paid to surrogates through the clinic materially improve their lives rather than serving only as wages and profit to the clinic. Whereas surrogates may understand surrogacy in terms of religion or as otherwise outside of market logics.

Biogenetic Parenthood: Kinship and the Work of Surrogacy

Hanging on the wall of the director's office in the small but growing Manushi clinic is a multimedia work commissioned by the clinic's director. A line of soft abstract shapes representing the salwar chemise-clad pregnant bodies and covered heads of six women arcs around a central and taller abstracted female figure dressed in white. A group of staff explained to me that the central figure in white represents the director, Dr. Bhakta, herself. Her arms are outstretched to encompass the group of women, whose most distinguishing features are their exaggerated wombs, marked as embossed circles with a centered fetal-imprint pressed into the plastic material of their bodily forms. According to one staff member, the piece is meant to portray the director's vision of the clinic's surrogacy practice as a form of altruism and care for the women who become commercial surrogates, and the image is a way to signpost this vision to commissioning parents who visit the clinic. The image also represents the pregnant body as imagined through the discourse of the medicalized body, where the uterus is an empty and un-utilized space. The artistic representation draws attention to the central importance of the once-empty uterus. Now filled, the womb marks the service being performed by the surrogates and reflects the primary way that the clinic encourages potential and active surrogates themselves to approach gestational surrogacy as a service.

As reproductive technologies and associated medical discourse developed primarily in advanced capitalist countries have traveled to India, they have been accompanied by co-constituting Euro-American notions of kinship as biogenetically based (Inhorn and Birenbaum-Carmeli 2008). One of the outcomes of the way that medical discourse about reproductive technologies, through this linking of kinship and biogenetics, distances actual individualized bodies from the biology of reproduction, is that it creates a framework for commissioning parents, doctors, and surrogates to imagine the act of gestating a child as a paid occupation in which a service (gestation and childbirth) is exchanged for a fee. The exchange is not limited to these terms, but the way that medical discourse isolates the reproductive body and gametes from the social context in which they originated allows for gestational surrogacy to be conceived of as a form of paid work or service by participants.

Most of the women who come to the Manushi clinic come from at least an hour's bus ride away, and generally find out about the opportunity through friends or family. According to the clinic's guidelines, a potential surrogate must be married with at least one child and have permission from her husband to be eligible. Once pregnant, surrogates are highly encouraged to live in designated housing near the clinic where they can rest instead of working and providing care to their families. This arrangement also allows for surveillance by clinic staff. Their husbands, sometimes accompanied by children, come to visit them in these hostels during the weekends. Most surrogates hide their participation from extended family and sometimes even their own children because of the associated stigma.

The overall surrogacy process at this clinic costs clients roughly 20,000 dollars, depending on whether or not they use donor eggs and how many in vitro fertilization cycles are necessary to accomplish a pregnancy. The clinic mandates that embryos be created using either the intended mother's ova or those of a donor, but never those of the gestational surrogate. Egg donors and surrogates are selected by the director rather than by the commissioning parents. After an initial interview, there is usually little contact between surrogate mothers and intended parents. The relationship between the intended parents and their surrogate is almost always completely mediated by the clinic staff. Clients who come to this clinic from abroad to hire surrogates cite a number of reasons for their decision, including the desire for a child who shares genetic material with one or both parents, the comparatively high cost and administrative complexity of domestic and international adoption, and because in some cases, the clients' home countries do not allow surrogacy or only allow it under limited circumstances such as in noncommercial arrangements. The Manushi clinic only accepts client couples for surrogacy when they are heterosexual, and when the woman cannot physically support a pregnancy herself. The clinic has suspended this first rule in the case of a small number of male single-parent clients, and it is conceivable that these individuals might be part of nonheterosexual family formations. The latter rule is meant to insure that the clinic is only arranging surrogacy when it is "medically necessary" and to prevent clients from using surrogates to avoid pregnancy.

Becoming a Surrogate Mother

The Manushi clinic started out as an Obstetrics and Gynecology clinic that offered IVF, where embryos created outside the body are transferred to a woman's womb for gestation. After the clinic's first successful surrogacy case and the resultant media coverage, demand led the clinic to first hire recruited surrogates, and then later self-referred surrogates. Dr. Naina Patel, director of the clinic, matches international clients with surrogate mothers based on a variety of factors including the age of gestational and biological mothers. When the client herself does not have viable eggs, eggs from Indian donors are used, and this particular clinic stipulates that the surrogate and the donor must be separate individuals. This policy is meant to insure that the surrogate mother has no genetic claim on the child and to discourage emotional attachment to the child after it is born.

After an initial interview, there is usually little contact between surrogate mothers and intended parents. The relationship between the intended parents and their surrogate mother is almost always completely mediated by the clinic staff. US clients to whom I spoke about this practice noted that the doctors explained to them that this arrangement was in their best interest, as the surrogates almost never speak English, and the clients rarely speak Hindi or Gujarati. When the clients do speak one of these Indian languages, such as with nonresident Indian clients, there can be long-distance phone communication.

Surrogate mothers are highly encouraged to live in designated hostels near the clinic where they can rest instead of working and providing care to their families. Their families visit them in the hostels from homes outside the town of Anand. The two hostels offer computer, English language, and sewing courses, and have a cook who prepares food for the women. Counseling is available from the hostel manager, who is a former surrogate herself, as well as from other clinic staff who have been surrogates. Surrogates receive a fee of roughly 6000 dollars, which can be the equivalent of up to 9 years of their regular family income from their own or their husband's manual labor. The overall surrogacy process at this clinic costs clients about $20,000, in comparison to the roughly $100,000 it costs in the United States.

Most of the clients who come to India to hire surrogates, and all of the clients at the Manushi clinic, are heterosexual couples where the intended mother cannot carry a fetus to term herself. In this sense, the clients require a surrogate mother in order to create a child based on their own complete or partial genetic material. Some of the clients' home countries do not allow surrogacy or only allow it under limited circumstances, such as in noncommercial arrangements. Others come to India because they cannot or do not wish to pay the substantially higher cost for surrogacy in their home countries. In this way, ARTs simultaneously create the possibility of a biological child for couples who do not have the ability to produce one on their own, and demand for surrogate mothers.

Through counseling and conversations with doctors, a surrogate is encouraged to think of her womb as a space she can rent out; the analogy surrogates I spoke to use is that the womb is like a spare room in a home, where someone else's baby will stay and grow. One of the doctors at the clinic described the approach of clinic staff this way:

> "[we] try to explain to them that what you are doing, you are doing for someone else, whatever money or gifts they give you. The emotional attachment is going to be there, but they understand one thing, even if they are not educated that much, which is that we have to give the child back to the parents. That's one of the most important things, and we haven't had any case otherwise."

In discussing the anticipation of parting with the infant upon its birth, a number of the women working as surrogates explained independently that since the baby wouldn't look like her, she wouldn't feel a bond with it. This explanation is used by doctors to guide surrogates in thinking of the child as not their own. Despite this coaching and the understanding that the babies are not theirs, women who had already delivered did say they missed the infants after they left India and hoped to hear about their development, receive pictures of the children, and maintain a connection to these families.

The prominent narrative of the distance between a gestational surrogate and the eventual infant she will deliver as an inevitable result of the genetic distance between the two is a product of a western medical discourse of the body and biogenetics of parenthood. Emily Martin has observed the ways that the medical gaze, particularly as administered through visual technologies like ultrasonography, enforces the Cartesian mind/body dualism and alienates pregnant women from the process of being pregnant. She has elaborated this as the obstetrician becoming a "mechanic" and the pregnant woman a "laborer" (Martin 2001, 57). As will be discussed in more detail in the next chapter, the relationship to and understanding of the womb as a separable body part from the woman's whole body and from herself as a subject, and hence of the baby as a guest that is not part of her body, is a product of an understanding of the body and self which must be naturalized for the women acting as surrogates, and allows participants to understand gestation as a form of paid work. At the same time, this does not exhaust the meaning of how surrogates understand their social relations and even kinship relations with commissioning parents and the infant they bear, as Amrita Pande's recent study of surrogates and kinship at a fertility clinic in Gujarat reveals (Pande 2009a).

Women who were currently working as surrogates explained the need for secrecy that many felt as resulting from the fact that people in their communities would not understand that she had not had sexual relations in order to conceive, and therefore surrogacy would not be accepted as an altruistic act or as valid employment. At the same time, everyone I spoke to expressed conviction that carrying another person's child as a surrogate was not compromising any moral standards around sexuality, a trend which is supported by Amrita Pande's observations of commercial surrogacy in India (Pande 2009b). This conviction is at least partially the result of the coaching in the process and meaning of conception and childbirth received through the clinic's explanations of how surrogacy makes a fetus but not a mother from the surrogate. These explanations are based on the western medical understanding of the genetic basis of parenthood, though whether or not the surrogate mothers themselves fully accept their role within these terms is not clear in their versions of the clinic's narrative of how surrogacy works, and is challenged by the way that surrogates explain their role in terms of the divine, discussed below.

In addition to the intervention of western medical discourses of the body and biogenetic parenthood, it is the availability of women in India as surrogates, through both economic necessity and the lack of formal regulation, that makes transnational Indian surrogacy possible. Barbara Katz Rothman has argued that in the United States, discourse about surrogacy figures the surrogate's womb as property to use as she sees fit, and the fetus as property belonging to the intended parent (2000, 29). This discourse has traveled with the technologies involved in surrogacy, so that the understanding of procreation and parenthood that surrogate mothers are taught includes the figuring of the womb as a place to rent out for use by someone else's infant. The technologies that define and separate the roles of egg donor, intended mother, and gestational mother, in combination with the patriarchal discourse of infant-as-property, work with the commodifying logics of capitalist culture to objectify the work of gestation and the fetus so that they can participate as commodities in the transnational surrogacy industry. Even so, it is essential to note that this is not the primary economy to which women working as surrogates describe their labor as contributing. While women readily acknowledge that it is the demands of material circumstances that impel them to take up this otherwise undesirable work, many women also described their role of a surrogate in terms of an altruistic, or even divine, economy.

Altruism and the Divine

In the discussion and description of what it is like to be a part of transnational surrogacy arrangements in this clinic, doctors, surrogates, and commissioning parents all described their interest and actions as at least partially if not primarily motivated by altruism. In the context of clinic staff, this discourse took the form of a general narrative of the clinic's project of social work: rehabilitating women who take on surrogacy into more disciplined, self-sufficient, and professionalized workers, and helping childless couples from around the world build their families. Intended parents also described the opportunity to help needy women working as surrogates as part of the benefit of hiring a surrogate in India rather than in their home countries. In the context of how surrogates describe their participation, carrying a child for a couple without children is described in empathetic and spiritual terms as an opportunity to provide something that is usually the domain of a godly gift.

Many of the surrogate mothers I spoke to, all of whom were Hindu or Christian, emphasized a feeling that they were doing something great, often in religious language of being like a god, or being able to give a gift to an infertile couple that is a gift usually given only by god.[2] Most were usually quick to then include the doctors as part of this ability to provide, but the emphasis was on their own power to give. Those who spoke to this topic emphasized that this exalted aspect of their actions was much more important than the money aspect, and in fact was their primary motivation. At the same time, when I asked one former surrogate mother how she would feel if one of her daughters wanted to be a surrogate when she was older, her reply was immediate and negative: she explained that the whole reason she herself undertook a surrogacy was so that her children could become educated and wouldn't have to do such things, and that she would not want her daughters to experience that pain. I have to assume that she meant a certain experience of pain, both physical and emotional, that exists in surrogacy but not in carrying and birthing one's own child. Her comments also suggest that despite the narrative of the gift, which mediates the economic transactions within surrogacy by putting them in the realm of voluntary exchange and altruism, surrogacy is a type of work that is not desirable except when economically necessary.

The turn to the divine within these narratives can offer an alternative explanation of the meaning of surrogacy in a frame that is not limited to the medical discourse of the body and biogenetic parenthood. In the context of the clinic, it marks both a woman's powerful role as a surrogate, and signifies the value of the outcome of producing a child for a childless couple in nonmonetary terms. For the reader and scholar who does not originate from within the communities where the women working as surrogates reside, this mode of understanding and relating surrogacy could suggest a way to approach the significance of this act in terms beyond those of labor and economics. It could also provide a way to bridge potential gaps in women's understanding of the clinical explanation of surrogacy as a reproductive technology, which the doctors describe again and again to surrogates in a very basic way as a mode of recruitment. This includes the explanation of how in vitro fertilization works, where an infant is conceived without sexual relations, ultimately leading to the birth of child who "does not look like you." The discourse of the divine aspects of surrogacy suggests alternate ways that surrogacy might be imagined and have value that don't translate to the genetic definition of a biological parent, and don't necessarily circulate within the economic logic of surrogacy as technologically mediated "women's work" in the global economy.

Medicine, the Body, and Power in Decolonial India

Is the process of becoming biological workers (Vora 2009a) for women who participate in commercial surrogacy a process of neoliberal subject-making that echoes processes in the colonial period, when western medical discourse functioned as part of European experiments with modernity in their colonies (Prakash 1999, 13)? The precise answer cannot be determined without extensive research over time, and in fact might need to be written and theorized in part by the surrogates themselves. At the least, the context of commercial surrogacy in India raises fascinating questions that continue observations about the role of medical discourse, the body, and power made since the time of British colonial rule.

Putting Indian commercial surrogacy in the context of the scholarship on the role of western medicine in the colonial period suggests that the body has been and remains an independent signifier and site of subaltern modes of being even in the clinic, and even when surrogates themselves at least partially reproduce and utilize the rhetoric of the western medicalized body. As discussed in Chapter 2, the work of David Arnold and Gyan Prakash tracks the entanglements of empire, economics, science, power, and the formations of culture and subjectivity during British colonial rule. In his work on epidemic disease in the 19th-century India, David Arnold has demonstrated how the body, and particularly the Indian colonial body, has historically been a site of colonization and conquest (1988, 392, 1993, 15). This observation points to the corporeality of the British colonial project in India, but also yields the body and discourse about the body as sites for contestations of power in Indian history. Indian transnational surrogacy provides an important lens to view ways that specific technologies, instruments of measure and examination, and materializations of the body continue to manifest contested power and subjectivities within medicine as an institution and a global market. For example, the re-formulation of the surrogates' bodies as empty spaces that can be cultivated to re-produce western society and western lives recapitulates the colonial epistemology of land as property, where resources, including native labor, were used to sustain the metropole. This contemporary racialized and gendered political economic relationship rests upon a biopolitical order undergirded by access to technology, in this case reproductive technology.

As political and economic structures in India have been re-organized through independence and later neoliberalization, these precedents have been recast in interesting ways that share continuity with what Arnold observed in the 19th-century colonial structures of power and governance. We can see evidence of the effort to create neoliberal subjects in the coaching of surrogates into a particular relationship to their body and its abstraction through the medical gaze into parts with specific utility to the market, and through the process of imagining surrogates as workers through the alienation of pregnant women from the process of pregnancy encouraged by medical discourse and technology. In Chapter 3, I point to the dimensions of transnational Indian commercial surrogacy that operate as a neoliberalized form of reproductive labor, and specifically as a form of biological labor, I aim to contribute to a feminist analysis of the bioeconomy called for by Catherine Waldby and Melinda Cooper in their discussion of human oocyte vending. They describe such labor as unrecognized as such, due to the fact that it is comprised of giving clinics access to the productivity of women's bodies, rather than consisting of specific tasks (59). They also note a larger dynamic in the global economy for this "clinical labor (Ibid.)," which when taken together with scholarship on the trade in human organs (Scheper-Hughes 2001; Cohen 2001) and clinical trial subjects (Petryna 2006; Sundar Rajan 2006), points to the outsourcing of the clinical labor with the highest risk and undesirability to populations in the Global South (59–60). Masao Miyoshi (1993) has pointed out how transnational corporations, central global neoliberalizing forces, have extended and rearticulated colonialism, and by looking at the global market for biological labor (Vora 2009b), and clinical labor (Cooper and Waldby 2014), it would seem that neoliberal logics organizing labor markets similarly rearticulate colonial logics.

The meaning of surrogacy to different participants is complicated by their different understanding of the process itself, as well as different understandings, experience, and expectations of the social relations involved and generated in the clinic. This is taken up in Chapters 3 and 4. Gestational surrogates at the Manushi clinic are subjected to the medical gaze in a way that they have not been in prior pregnancies, and are encouraged by clinic staff to see their own bodies and pregnancies through the medical gaze in order to work toward separating surrogacy from noncommercial gestation, and to see surrogacy as a way to improve their lives materially through the financial opportunity it provides. Yet surrogates maintain that the divine aspects of their participation outweigh material considerations. The Manushi clinic's surrogacy practice proves to be a valuable lens for examining the intersection of reproductive technologies, the worldviews and self-understandings of various participants, as well as the general neoliberal disciplining of biological reproduction as a form of labor.

Notes

1 All identifying details of names and locations have been altered.
2 The vast majority of surrogates describe themselves as Hindu, and though there have been some Christian surrogates, the clinic directors report that they have only had one or two Muslim women who inquired about the process of becoming a surrogate, and explained this by saying that they don't often have Muslim women who are interested for reasons of spiritual beliefs about the integrity of the body. This can also be attributed to the fact that the clinic is located in an area with rather high Hindu-Muslim communal tensions, and the clinic directors are Hindu; their word of mouth recruiting strategy only reaches people who are already connected with the clinic or with past surrogates and as such would tend to be Hindu or Christian as well.

Works Cited

Arnold, David. (1988). *Colonizing the Body*. Berkeley and Los Angeles: University of California Press.

Arnold, Davis. (1993). "Touching the Body: Perspectives on the Indian Plague," in *Selected Subaltern Studies*, Ranajit Guha and Gayatri Chakravorty Spivak, eds. New York: Oxford University Press, pp. 391–426.

Bharadwaj, A. (2000). "How Some Indian Baby Makers are Made: Media Narratives and Assisted Conception in India," *Anthropology & Medicine*, 7: 63–78.

Cohen, Lawrence. (2001). "The Other Kidney: Biopolitics Beyond Recognition," *Body and Society*, 7(2–3): 9–29.

Colen, S. (1995). "'Like a Mother to Them': Stratified Reproduction and West Indian Childcare Workers and Employers in New York," in *Conceiving the New World Order: The Global Politics of Reproduction*, Faye Ginsburg and Rayna Rapp, eds. Berkeley: University of California Press, pp. 78–102.

Cooper, Melinda and Catherine Waldby. (2014). *Clinical Labor: Tissue Donors and Research Subjects in the Global Bioeconomy*. Durham, NC: Duke University Press.

Inhorn, Marcia C. and Aditya Bharadwaj. (2007). "Reproductively Disabled Lives: Infertility, Stigma, and Suffering in Egypt and India," in *Disability in Local and Global Worlds*, B. Ingstad and S.R. Whyte, eds. Berkeley: University of California Press, pp. 78–106.

Inhorn, Marcia C. and Daphna Birenbaum-Carmeli. (2008). "Assisted Reproductive Technologies and Culture Change," *Annual Review of Anthropology*, 37: 177–196.

Inhorn, Marcia C., R. Ceballa and R. Nachtigall. (2008). "Marginalized, Invisible, and Unwanted: American Minority Struggles with Infertility and Assisted Conception," in *Marginalised Reproduction: Ethnicity, Infertility and Assisted Conception*, N. Culley, N. Hudson and F. Van Rooij, eds. London: Earthscan.

Martin, Emily. (2001). *The Woman in the Body: A Cultural Analysis of Reproduction*. Boston: Beacon Press, p. 57.

Miyoshi, Masao. (1993). "A Borderless World? From Colonialism to Transnationalism and the Decline of the Nation-State," *Critical Inquiry*, 19(4): 725–751.

Pande, Amrita. (2009a). "It May Be Her Eggs but It Is My Blood: Surrogates and Everyday Forms of Kinship in India," *Qualitative Sociology*, 32(4): 379–397.

Pande, Amrita. (2009b). "Not an Angel, Not a Whore: Surrogates as Dirty Workers in India," *Indian Journal of Gender Studies*, 16(2): 141–173.

Petryna, Adriana. (2006). "Globalizing Human Subjects Research," in *Global Pharmaceuticals: Ethics, Markets, Practices*, Adriana Petryna, Andrew Lakoff and Arthur Kleinman, eds. Durham, NC: Duke University Press.

Prakash, Gyan. (1999). *Another Reason: Science and the Imagination of Modern India*. Princeton, NJ: Princeton University Press.

Rothman, B. Katz. (2000). *Recreating Motherhood*. New Brunswick, NJ: Rutgers University Press, p. 29.

Scheper-Hughes, Nancy. (2001). "Commodity Fetishism in Organs Trafficking," *Body and Society*, 7(2–3): 31–62.

Spar, Debora. (2006). *The Baby Business: How Money, Science, and Politics Drive the Commerce of Conception*. Boston: Harvard Business School Press.

Sundar Rajan, Kaushik. (2006). *Biocapital: The Constitution of Postgenomic Life*. Durham, NC: Duke University Press, 2006.

Vora, Kalindi. (2009a). "Indian Transnational Surrogacy and the Commodification of Vital Energy," *Subjectivities*, 28(1): 266–278.

Vora, Kalindi. (2009b). "Other's Organs and the Production of Life: South Asian Domestic Labor and Human Kidneys," *Postmodern Culture*, 19(1).

Waldby, Catherine and Melinda Cooper. (2008). "The Biopolitics of Reproduction," *Australian Feminist Studies*, 23.

3

INDIAN TRANSNATIONAL SURROGACY AND THE COMMODIFICATION OF VITAL ENERGY

Assisted reproductive technologies (ARTs) allow women to sell the service of gestating a fetus but maintain little or no claim to the product of that labor: the child itself. In the context of transnational Indian surrogacy, this situation is exacerbated by the physical and cultural distance between intended parents and surrogates. The productive nature of the care and nurturing provided through the work of mothering becomes more visible when viewed though the commodification of commercial surrogacy. Once commodified, this work of care also becomes subject to the alienation of capitalist relations, which invites us to investigate the social and economic implications of the work of mothering in surrogacy. I argue that care and nurture in transnational Indian surrogacy invest human vital energy as a form of value directly into other human beings, through the biological and affective labor involved in surrogate work, thereby supporting the lives of those individuals, families, and societies that consume this energy.

In early 2015, the Indian government had no active legislation around commercial surrogacy, and for this reason studying the practices at individual fertility clinics with surrogacy services was important because each clinic decided to what extent they follow the existing guidelines for ART clinics.[1] Until the ban of transnational surrogacy arrangements at the end of 2015, draft legislation remained under consideration in the Indian parliament in the form of the Draft Assisted Reproductive Technologies (Regulation) Bill and Rules. It was proposed in late 2008, and was redrafted several times to meet demands by different interest groups in India, while also promoting conditions that support the market. By observing the particular policies at the pseudonymous Manushi clinic, I was able to view firsthand the way that the social relations entailed by surrogacy agreements and the necessary financial arrangements are organized. The goal of this essay is to raise preliminary theoretical questions arising from the context of gestation and childbirth as forms of labor in Indian surrogacy. After outlining the surrogacy process at the clinic I visited, I will look at how commercial surrogacy in India relies on a western medical understanding of the body that has constructed the uterus as surplus, and a genetics-based model of parentage

DOI: 10.4324/9781003353362-3

that emphasizes a connection between the intended parents and fetus and a distance between the surrogate and the guest-fetus. After this, I will briefly discuss some of the ways that social and financial exchange occurs between surrogates and intended parents both inside and outside the relationship established by the clinic. I will conclude by suggesting how the "surplus" wombs of the Indian women who become surrogates fit into a broader context of how life becomes abstracted as a commodity form.

In order to understand commercial surrogacy as work, I suggest the frameworks of affective and biological labor to describe the work of self-care, nurture, and gestation performed by the surrogate toward herself and the fetus she carries. Because the consumers and producers of the biological and affective labor commodified in commercial surrogacy are marked by differentials of class, race, and gender, Indian transnational surrogacy reproduces a disparity between where this value is extracted and where it is invested. This puts transnational Indian surrogacy into conversation with similar trends in surrogacy in other locations (Ragone 1994; Sandelowski 1993; Teman 2010) and with literature on organ selling (Cohen 2001; Scheper-Hughes 2001), and maids, nannies, and domestic workers (Gamburd 2000; Ismail 1999; Parreñas 2001; Tadiar 2004; Vora 2009). These studies point to the ways intersections of race, class, gender, and nationality position certain subjects as more appropriate for devalued service work than others. Race and gender also operate in the global political economy to make some bodies more economically useful as biological entities than as the source of labor, and to render some subjects seemingly more appropriate for reorganization as biological laborers than others (Vora 2009).

Becoming a Surrogate

When working as a surrogate becomes an option in a given location in India, women from that region begin to understand surrogacy as a way to establish economic security and self-recruit to approach reproductive clinics. Women interested in working as surrogates—most often day-laborers from rural communities with a middle school- or high school-equivalent education—arrive for an interview with clinic staff who give them a basic understanding of IVF. This is meant to help them both to understand that surrogacy does not involve their bodies sexually, and also to encourage them to emotionally distance themselves from the fetus and the child they will deliver. Through counseling and conversation, medical personnel encourage surrogates to see themselves as gestation-providers whose only link to the fetus is the renting of a womb imagined as an empty and otherwise unproductive space. This formulation of surrogacy and pregnancy makes possible the commodification of the womb and the disaggregation of the work of mothering into distinct affective and biological components—necessary conditions for the transnational distribution of this work.

The analogy most surrogates use to explain what they are doing is that the womb is like a spare room in a home, where someone else's baby will stay and grow. The baby is a guest—separable from rather than part of the woman's whole body, and thus distinct from the surrogate as a subject. The relationship each woman develops with her womb and the fetus it supports is thus (at least partially) constructed from conceptions of the body and promoted by medical staff, and linked to the ways in which western medical culture makes sense of kinship through ARTs. Notions of kinship deriving from these technologies are actively taught to the surrogates at the clinic to a degree that surrogate mothers eventually seem to accept these notions, at least as far as they allow them to go through with surrogacy.

ARTs have made it possible to disaggregate the work of motherhood into (1) the provision of an ovum and gestation a fetus, and (2) the work and care of child-rearing and what Charis Thomson calls "procreative intent," and then to differentially value these kinds of labor and distribute them across class and national lines. At the same time, however, a number of surrogates describe expectations of future responsibility on the part of the client to the surrogate and her family that lie outside the surrogate's fees and correspond to local notions of familial duty, implying that their acceptance of the logic put forward by medical staff is far from complete, and their understanding of mothering work as disaggregated may not be absolute.

Affective and Biological Labor

Affective labor, or the work of care and attention performed by people such as customer service agents, maids, and nannies, produces commodities of comfort, nurture and security that are not physical objects, yet are consumed in a way that causes others to feel better and more valuable. These "feelings" are necessities that are essential to human life and the ability to imagine oneself or one's community as having a viable future. As the products of affective work in India are often exported and consumed by citizens of wealthier nations, the vital energy contained in them is transmitted from the individuals and communities where it is produced to clients overseas. The concept of affective labor comes out of the scholarship of materialist and socialist feminists beginning in the 1970s and continuing to the present, including formulations of emotional labor (Hochschild 1985), the international division of care (Parreñas 2001), and outlawed (affective) necessities (Hennessy 2000). This scholarship examines the role of domestic labor, sex work, and emotional work in capitalist economies.

The concept of biological labor points to the commodification of biological bodily capacities that are sold in addition to or instead of more recognizable forms of work performed by the body. These capacities range from the production of unique DNA sequences and other biological information to the production of bodily tissues and parts such as blood and organs. In the context of commercial surrogacy, the surrogate mother's service of gestating the embryo and fetus is a form of biological labor. Since this service doesn't require the type of visible intention and effort that other forms of service work might entail, I refer to it as biological labor to clearly mark the intention and the cost in vitality that would be apparent in other forms of work.

Both biological and affective commodities produced by these types of labor are alienated through intertwined cultural and technological processes, expanding the realms of commodification as well as increasing the depth of commodification into the subject. The capitalist subject was first described by Marx as "he" who was alienated from access to land and therefore the means of production, who therefore had to sell his labor to factory owners who still had access to the means of production. The identification of affective and biological labor points to a change in the subject of capitalist production. This subject participates in not only a global commodification of labor power, but also a global organization of affective and biological production. Such production requires the subject to discipline the emotions and the self-care of the body as commodified activities within a globalized system of production. Since the 1970s, feminist materialists have recognized that there is more to capitalist production than what is visible in waged labor. For example, they were the first to point out that domestic labor in the worker's home was not calculated in the wage-earner's remunerations. The concept of biological labor continues this practice in making visible the feminized labor of commercial surrogacy.

The self-care of surrogates while they are carrying a guest fetus provides an example of how affective and biological labor plays a role in the transmission of value as vital energy. Bhumika,[1] a young woman from a town 20 km away from the clinic I visited who was 5 months pregnant as a surrogate mother when we spoke, illustrated this to me when she explained that she had already given birth to two children of her own, and that she had not taken nearly as much care or thought toward herself during those pregnancies as she was currently. For more than half of each of those pregnancies she had been employed in cleaning other people's houses. As a surrogate, she paid careful attention to the condition of the pregnancy, mentioning, for example, that she was eating much better and taking more rest. Like the other surrogates working with this clinic, she had signed an agreement that she would receive trimesterly maintenance stipends as long as she was pregnant, and would only receive her fee if she successfully completed her pregnancy. She also mentioned that she did not have the attention of a doctor in her previous pregnancies, no less the kind of technologically mediated care she was receiving as the gestational surrogate to a US couple. Intended parents, or clients, pay fees for the room and board of the surrogate separately from the medical expenses and fees for the surrogacy. Bhumika, like many surrogates at this clinic, was staying apart from her family in the surrogate housing that serves the clinic for the course of her pregnancy.

The clients I spoke to about this topic said they were reassured by the hostel arrangements for their surrogates, as this meant that they were close to good medical care and would eat clean, nutritious food and avoid heavy work that might endanger the pregnancy. These types of interactions are simultaneously acts of care, for the surrogate by her clients, and by the surrogate for the fetus and herself, as well as economic acts that protect the fetus and future child as a commodity and the surrogate's well-being as the only worker who can produce that commodity through her biological labor.

The Surrogacy Process

Most of the clients who come to India to hire surrogates are heterosexual couples in which the intended mother is unable to carry a fetus to term; in the clinic where I was based, these were stipulated conditions of eligibility. In some cases clients come to India because their home countries do not allow surrogacy or only allow it under limited circumstances, such as in noncommercial arrangements. Other would be parents come to India because they cannot or do not wish to pay the substantially higher cost for surrogacy in their home countries. The clients who seek out a surrogate mother are often motivated by the wish to create a child based on their own complete or partial genetic material. ARTs simultaneously create the possibility of a biological child for couples who do not have the ability to produce one without outside intervention, and they create the need for surrogate mothers.

The clinic I observed began as an Obstetrics and Gynecology clinic that also offered in vitro fertilization (IVF), a process in which embryos created outside the body are transferred to a woman's womb for gestation. Over time, the clinic has shifted its focus to fertility and surrogacy services. The director of the clinic matches international clients with surrogate mothers based on a variety of factors including the ages of gestational and biological mothers. When the client herself does not have viable eggs, eggs from Indian donors are used. At this particular clinic, they stipulate that the surrogate and the donor must be separate individuals to ensure that the surrogate mother has no genetic claim on the child and to discourage her emotional attachment to the child after its birth.

After an initial interview, there is usually little contact between surrogate mothers and intended parents. The relationship between the intended parents and their surrogates during gestation is almost always completely mediated by the clinic staff. US clients to whom I spoke about this practice noted that the doctors explained to them that this arrangement was in their best interest, as the surrogates almost never speak English, and the clients rarely speak Hindi or regional languages. When the clients do speak one of these Indian languages, such as with nonresident Indian clients, there can be long-distance phone communication after the initial meeting. For the most part, however, such communication is limited, leaving little opportunity for bonding between surrogates and their clients.

Surrogate mothers are highly encouraged to live in designated housing near the clinic where they can rest instead of working and providing care to their families, and where they remain under watch by clinic staff. Their families visit them from homes outside the town where the clinic is located. The two hostels offer computer, English language, and sewing courses, and have a cook who prepares food for the women. Counseling is available from the house manager, who is a former surrogate herself, as well as from other clinic staff who have been surrogates. Surrogates receive a fee of between $6000 and $7000, which can be the equivalent of up to 9 years of their regular family income from their own or their husband's work. The overall surrogacy process at this clinic costs clients around $20,000, in comparison to the roughly $100,000 it costs in the United States.

Constructing the Empty Womb

Following the work of anthropologists Rayna Rapp and Emily Martin, who have examined the ways that technology and the cultural realities of gendered embodiment are co-constituted, I want to examine two constructions in commercial Indian surrogacy: the so-called empty uterus of the would-be surrogate, and the surrogate's role as a service-provider rather than a parent. Feminist scholars and anthropologists have established that medical and particularly visual technologies have altered the way that women understand and relate to their bodies (see also Kevles 1998; Stabile 1998). The medical construction of the pregnant body becomes visible in my fieldwork as women who want to be surrogates are encouraged by doctors to think of their bodies through the western medical model, where the body operates like a machine composed of parts and exists largely separate from the self. A surrogate is seen as a service provider rather than a parent through the western medical understanding of parenthood as based purely in biology, so that the woman who is the source of the egg or the woman who is the wife of the source of the sperm is the mother of the child; the woman who gives birth to the child is not necessarily a member of the mother–child pair. As I will explain, this notion of parenthood as mediated by technology is very difficult to explain to members of some surrogates' communities.

One of the surrogate mothers with whom I spoke was Durga, a 24-year-old mother of one from a town an hour away from the clinic who had recently been hired as a surrogate. When I spoke to her, she had just undergone an attempt at implantation with an embryo created from the egg and sperm of a Canadian couple. Durga's husband had come with her for the embryo transfer and waited with her to hear the result. She was scheduled to rest there in a bed in one of the clinic's common rooms until she heard if she had become pregnant, waiting along with four other women in a similar condition. Durga explained how she decided to become a surrogate: "I have a friend in my neighborhood who was a surrogate [for this clinic], and she told me about this opportunity. She explained to me that my womb is like an extra room in a house that I don't need, and can be rented out. The baby stays there for nine months, so it has a place to grow, but it is not your baby."

Durga's explanation of the physical process and meaning of gestational surrogacy, where the womb can be isolated within a woman's body and from herself and is imagined as an empty space in which a guest fetus will temporarily reside, reflects one of the primary conditions of possibility for the growth of transnational surrogacy in India. Through a narrative of procreation with IVF that separates the body producing the baby from genetic reproduction, and technologies that free fertilization and gestation from being tied to a single biological individual, the womb can be imagined as a surplus part whose use a woman can sell without compromising her cultural values.

The directors of the clinic are careful to explain to potential surrogates how the technology of IVF will allow them to temporarily house a baby that is actually someone else's child. In the case of surrogacy at this clinic, there is an effort to train women into a new understanding of their bodies that allows them to conceive of their uterus as an empty space that is not being used, and therefore can be hired out. This training also situates them in a previously unimagined relationship (or lack of relationship) to the child they will bear. The clinic's director told me how it is necessary for her to explain how surrogacy works to women interested in becoming surrogates, both to assure them that there is nothing sexual involved, as well as to guide them into the desired understanding of their relation to the child they will bear. The majority of women who are interested in becoming surrogates are unfamiliar with the technologies involved in conception through IVF. Instead of attempting to explain this technologically mediated mode of understanding the body and reproduction, most surrogates choose to hide their pregnancies from their extended families and communities—a decision which also makes staying in the sponsored housing more appealing. When I talked to surrogates about the need for secrecy, most of them felt since people in their communities were unfamiliar with IVF, they would not understand that the surrogate's body had not been involved sexually in the conception process. This misunderstanding would prevent the surrogacy from being accepted. Counseling and schooling from doctors at the clinic gives surrogates a basic understanding of IVF that allows them to keep their sense of propriety around reproduction and sexuality intact, and emphasizes the privileging of genetic parentage over the mother who births the child to encourage surrogate mothers to see themselves as distinct from the intended mother of the child. That is, the surrogate is encouraged to see herself as a subject of service work, not as what is being distinguished as the subject who is the mother of the child.

Despite the coaching in the understanding that the infants are not theirs, the former surrogates I spoke with did say that they missed the children after they left India and hoped to hear about their development and receive pictures. Some surrogates indicated the hope of an ongoing relationship with the intended parents that would continue to benefit themselves and their families in the future. For example, some surrogates have tried to establish pseudo-kinship relations of the patron and client through the Indian cultural model of duty, where the clients have a duty toward the surrogate mother after the child is given to them, and even though she makes no claim on the child, the surrogate might feel she can make a claim on the clients as patrons.[2] These observations indicate that while the genetic narrative may render surrogacy and the inevitable alienation from the child emotionally manageable, it certainly does not fully account for the lived experience of surrogacy or understanding of kinship held by those who participate; though the surrogate is disciplined away from being a parental subject, she may become a subject of other types of kinship. An important area for further research is in the ways that surrogates understand their bodies and pregnancy before they encounter surrogates and the clinic staff, and how they regard their relationship to the fetus during gestation and after delivery.

The medicalized version of the surrogate's body depends on an acceptance of the separation of body and self, and the concept of the body as a machine that works in parts, so that the uterus becomes just an empty space which is not being used when a woman is not pregnant. This construction of the pregnant body also allows the surrogate to see her participation as a form of work or employment, and to see her relation to the fetus/child as temporary and different from that of a parent. A parent, in turn, is defined as someone who has a biological, and specifically a genetic relationship to the fetus and child. However, as Helene Ragone and Charis Thompson have indicated, this construction of the biology of parenthood, where blood is transmitted through genes, comes apart in donor-egg IVF (Ragone 1994; Thompson 2005).

The technologies that divide the work and roles of the subject of mothering into egg donor, intended mother, and gestational mother also work with the commodifying logics of capitalist culture to objectify the mother and the fetus so that they can participate as commodities in the transnational surrogacy industry. The logic behind the genetic model of procreation that surrogate mothers are taught, where the womb becomes a place to rent out for use by someone else's baby, figures her womb as property to use as she sees fit, and the fetus as belonging to the intended parents. The womb is understood as a place where the egg and sperm develop into a baby, and therefore when the baby is born it is "given back" to its rightful owners (Katz Rothman 2000, 29). This understanding of their wombs as independent of their selves allows surrogates to distinguish surrogacy from infidelity, and to conceive of gestation as a form of work. These understandings combine with the technologies that isolate and disperse procreation in a way that allows for the alienation of the womb and mothering necessary for their commodification.

Investment in US Families

The medicalized body, and the distinction of social from "biological (in this case genetic) parenting" (Strathern 1992, 27–28), allows the women working as surrogates to see gestation as employment rather than kinship. It also creates an economic arrangement that transfers the benefit of the work of care, nurture and gestation provided by the surrogates to the family and community of the client parents. Despite the primary economic relationship, surrogates describe altruistic motivations as more important to them than financial motivations. Also, though the interactions between surrogates and clients are limited, relationships between them do exist, and these can exceed both the social and economic bounds of their relations as defined through capitalism and the clinic's surrogacy agreement.

Many of the surrogate mothers with whom I spoke, regardless of whether they were Hindu or Christian (no Muslim women were working as surrogates), emphasized a feeling that they were doing something great, often in religious language of being like a god, or being able to give a gift to an infertile couple that is a gift usually given only by god. Most were usually quick to then include the doctors as part of this ability to give, but the emphasis was on their own power to give. Those who spoke to this topic emphasized that this exalted aspect of their actions was much more important than the money aspect, and in fact was their primary motivation. At the same time, when I asked one former surrogate how she would feel if one of her daughters wanted to be a surrogate when she was older, her reply was immediate and negative. She explained that the whole reason she herself undertook surrogacy was so that her children could become educated and "wouldn't have to do such things." She said that she "would not want her daughters to experience that pain." I assume that she meant a certain experience of pain, both physical and emotional, that exists in surrogacy but not in the experience of carrying and birthing one's own child. Her comments also suggest that despite the narrative of the gift, which mediates the economic transactions within surrogacy by putting them in the realm of voluntary exchange and altruism, surrogacy is a type of work that is not desirable except when economically necessary.[3]

Intended parents sometimes express a feeling of duty or obligation to their surrogates beyond the required fee, which is usually between $5000 and $7000. I did hear of some intended parents writing to their surrogates and sending email and photos of the child in the first year, but most of the surrogates said they do not hear from their former clients very frequently, though they like to get these communications. Instead, the clients tend to feel a connection to "India" rather than to individual women. For example, one intended mother said she would tell her child that it was born in India, and hoped to bring the child to India to see where it was born. Intended parents' sense of duty and obligation, enacted through giving gifts and generally repressing the commodity nature of their exchange, has another important aspect. Such gifts are also described as compensating for the relatively low fees paid to surrogates, which both assuages the uncertainty and sometimes guilt that parents have about potentially exploiting the surrogates, as well as allowing them to feel that they are improving the lives of the surrogates.

One of the intended parents with whom I spoke, named David, arrived to the clinic from New York the same day as I did, and having never been to India, was keen to learn as much from me as he could. He was visibly nervous about the surrogacy process, and explained to me that his wife, who was over 45 years old, did not need to accompany him as he would be giving a semen sample later that day for use in creating an embryo with a donated egg. Other than the day's schedule, he had little knowledge of what the process would be for him during his 5 days at the clinic. During David's second day, one of the doctors invited me join him and David for a meeting during which David would have his first conversation with his assigned surrogate, Puja. After a couple of minutes of translating David's expressions of appreciation, the doctor left me to translate for David and Puja so that he could attend to other business. David asked me to tell Puja that he wanted her to come visit them in the United States in the future, and she responded enthusiastically. She then asked if she could bring her husband as well, and if they could find work in the United States. David became flustered and changed the topic to her health, asking if she was feeling well, and whether she was really comfortable with the idea of becoming a surrogate. Puja replied with self-assurance and professional formality, saying that she was absolutely comfortable with surrogacy. David then asked if she would mind if I took a picture of the two of them for his wife, and since she did not, I took a photo. David had no more questions, and after Puja left, David told me how unsettled he felt about his relationship to this woman who would be carrying his child, implying that something felt uncomfortably intimate about their relationship, though Puja was strictly professional during the interview. I didn't get to speak to Puja before she left the clinic, but at least her self-presentation was much more self-possessed and confident than David's. Later that day, David told me that after the doctor and I left the room, Puja asked him in English for additional money above the fees he was contracted to pay, and he said that he pretended he couldn't understand what she was asking.

David and his wife returned to the clinic to pick up their child 9 months later. They spoke to Puja by phone after they returned again to the United States, and she told them that she cried every night when she thought of how she would never see their baby again. David said that in response, he wrote her a letter telling her not to think that way. He mentioned to me that they were now wishing for siblings for their daughter using the same egg donor, but that they weren't sure that they could quote "put another surrogate through the process." David did not mention whether he intends to fulfill the wish he expressed to bring Puja and her family to the United States someday, though they clearly don't intend to work with Puja if they have another child. However, David is still sorting out his ongoing relationship to her and is wary of the affective impact of surrogacy on the surrogate's life.

Indian Surrogacy and Biocapital

The surrogate's self-care while pregnant and her nurturing of the fetus and newborn are forms of productive labor, that upon their consumption, yield immediate well-being and therefore future life opportunities for both the infant and its parents. As a number of scholars have noted, despite the fact that infertility is statistically more severe in resource-poor areas (Van Balen and Inhorn 2002; Inhorn 2003), assisted reproduction through advanced technology is only accessible to a global elite (Ginsburg and Rapp 1995). Articulating surrogacy as a form of work and identifying the value transmitted by the biological and affective commodities it produces—commodities that are invested directly by the work of care and nurture into an individual or community's life—enables us to view human lives as a site of the accumulation of the value produced by surrogates as workers. In the context of transnational surrogacy, this value is transmitted from lower resource communities to higher resource communities through the devaluing of this work as a result of its racialization and gendering.

Thinking about the work of gestation and nurture as forms of affective and biological labor in this way also points to the growing reach of biocapital as a paradigm. Sarah Franklin and Kaushik Sundar Rajan have used this concept to describe the rise of biological information as commodities and capital. I expand this formulation of biocapital to examine the commodification of the so-called empty uterus and the service of gestation. This more inclusive use of the framework of biocapital provides a way to understand, within a capitalist framework, how surrogacy can act as a form of productive labor through the investment of human vital energy directly into another person, family, and society to support their continued life.

The conditions of possibility for commercial surrogacy reflect the conditions that more generally allow for "life" to become an object of anthropological analysis (Rose 2006; Sundar Rajan 2006; Franklin 2001; Landecker 2007), and for life to gain the promissory quality that generates commercial markets around it. Commercial surrogacy in India, oriented primarily but not exclusively toward foreign clients, suggests that life in the specific sense of human reproduction, and even in the more abstract sense of the energy that the surrogate invests into the future life chances of the child produced, can carry exchange value, and that this impacts social relations through the very mode of production in commercial surrogacy. Such an analysis points to a transformation of capitalist production and exchange, not only in the context of production related to the biological sciences, but also to a paradigm shift in general where life, in many forms, becomes a commodity and carrier of value, a shift to biocapital.

The force of biocapital in the context of transnational Indian surrogacy becomes the compulsion to sell "life" as the body's long-term capacities (Waldby and Mitchell 2006, 23), and to sell vital energy in the form of gestation and nurture. In some ways this process is not vastly different from the history of selling labor power for a wage tracked by Marxist scholars, but the dominant currencies and epistemic understandings that shape this articulation of capital are different.

At the clinic I studied, the genetic model of parentage and the western medical conception of the body yield the pregnant body as a productive machine separate from the subject of the surrogate mother, and create the potential for her work of care, nurture, and gestation to become commodified. Transnational Indian surrogacy demonstrates some of the ways that reproductive technologies operate together with capitalist processes in increasing the density, or deepening interiority, of the commodification of labor within the subject. However, the social relations between doctors, surrogates, and intended parents also exceed the relations organized through capitalist exchange, and neither the surrogates nor their clients completely adhere to this relationship, occupying instead shifting positions of inter-relatedness.

Notes

1 All of the names and identifying details of those referred to in this essay have been changed.

2 For examples of the well-documented relationship of patron and client in India, see Beals 1974; Dube 1967; Lewis 1958; Pocock 1962.

3 See Amrita Pande's work for an elaboration of this sentiment among Indian surrogates.

Works Cited

Beals, A.R. (1974). *Village Life in South India*. Chicago, IL: Aldine.

Cohen, L. (2001). "The Other Kidney: Biopolitics Beyond Recognition," *Body and Society*, 7: 9–29.

Dube, S.C. (1967). *Indian Village*. New York: Harper Colophon Books.

Franklin, S. (2001). "Ethical Biocapital: New Strategies of Cell Culture," in *Remaking Life and Death*, S. Franklin and M. Lock, eds. Santa Fe and Oxford: School of American Research Press.

Gamburd, M. (2000). *The Kitchen Spoon's Handle: Transnationalism and Sri Lanka's Migrant Housemaids*. Ithaca, NY: Cornell University Press.

Ginsburg, F. and R. Rapp. (1995). "Introduction: Conceiving the New World Order," in *Conceiving the New World Order: The Global Politics of Reproduction*, F. Ginsburg and R. Rapp, eds. Berkeley, CA: University of California Press.

Hennessy, R. (2000). *Profit and Pleasure: Sexual Identities in Late Capitalism*. New York and London: Routledge.

Hochschild, A.R. (1985). *The Managed Heart: Commercialization of Intimate Feeling*. Berkeley: University of California Press.

Inhorn, M.C. (2003). "Global Infertility and the Globalization of New Reproductive Technologies: Illustrations from Egypt," *Social Science & Medicine*, 56: 1837–1851.

Ismail, M. (1999). "Maids in Space: Gendered Domestic Labor from Sri Lanka to the Middle East," in *Gender, Migration and Domestic Service*, J. Momsen, ed. London: Routledge.

Katz Rothman, B. (2000). *Recreating Motherhood*. New Brunswick, NJ: Rutgers University Press.

Kevles, B. (1998). *Naked to the Bone: Medical Imaging in the Twentieth Century*. Reading, MA: Addison-Wesley.

Landecker, H. (2007). *Culturing Life: How Cells Became Technologies*. Cambridge: Harvard University Press.

Lewis, O. (1958). *Village Life in Northern India*. New York: Random House, Vintage Books.

Martin, E. (2001). *The Woman in the Body: A Cultural Analysis of Reproduction*. Boston, MA: Beacon Press.

Marx, K., F. Engles and R.C. Tucker. (1978). *The Marx-Engels Reader*. New York: Norton.

Pande, A. (2010). "At Least I am Not Sleeping with Anyone: Resisting the Stigma of Commercial Surrogacy in India," *Feminist Studies*, 36(4).

Parreñas, R.S. (2000). "Migrant Filipina Domestic Labor and the International Division of Reproductive Labor," *Gender and Society*, 14(4): 560–580.

Parreñas, R.S. (2001). *Servants of Globalization: Women, Migration, and Domestic Work*. Stanford, CA: Stanford University Press.

Pocock, D.F. (1962). "Notes on Jajmani Relationships," *Contributions to Indian Sociology*, 6: 78–95.

Ragone, H. (1994). *Surrogate Motherhood: Conception in the Heart*. Boulder, CO and London: Westview Press.

Rapp, R. (1999). *Testing Women, Testing the Fetus: The Social Impact of Amniocentesis in America*. New York: Routledge.

Rose, N. (2006). *The Politics of Life Itself: Biomedicine, Power and Subjectivity in the Twenty-First Century*. Princeton: Princeton University Press.

Sandelowski, M. (1993). *With Child in Mind: Studies of the Personal Encounter with Infertility*. Philadelphia, PA: University of Pennsylvania Press.

Scheper-Hughes, N. (2001). "Commodity Fetishism in Organs Trafficking," *Body and Society*, 7(2–3): 32.

Stabile, C. (1998). "Shooting the Mother: Fetal Photography and the Politics of Disappearance," in *The Visible Woman: Imaging Technologies, Gender, and Science*,

P.A. Treichler, L. Cartwright and C. Penley, eds. New York: New York University Press.

Strathern, M. (1992). *After Nature: English Kinship in the Late Twentieth Century*. Cambridge: Cambridge University Press.

Sundar Rajan, K. (2006). *Biocapital: The Constitution of Postgenomic Life*. Durham, NC: Duke University Press.

Tadiar, N.X.M. (2004). *Fantasy Production: Sexual Economies and Other Philippine Consequences for the New World Order*. Hong Kong: Hong Kong University Press; London: Eurospan.

Teman, E. (2010). *Birthing a Mother: The Surrogate and the Body*. Berkeley, CA: University of California Press.

Thompson, C. (2005). *Making Parents: The Ontological Choreography of Reproductive Technologies*. Cambridge, MA: MIT Press.

Van Balen, F. and M.C. Inhorn. (2002). "Introduction—Interpreting Infertility: A View from the Social Sciences," in *Infertility Around the Globe: New Thinking on Childlessness, Gender, and Reproductive Technologies*, M.C. Inhorn and F. Van Balen, eds. Berkeley, CA: University of California Press, pp. 3–23.

Vora, K. (2009). "Others' Organs: South Asian Domestic Labor and the Kidney Trade," *Postmodern Culture*, 19: 1.

Waldby, C. and R. Mitchell. (2006). *Tissue Economies: Blood, Organs, and Cell Lines in Late Capitalism*. Durham, NC: Duke University Press.

4

LIMITS OF "LABOR"

Accounting for Affect and the Biological in Transnational Surrogacy and Service Work

Bharati is a typical call center agent in New Delhi. As a college graduate in urban India, she did not have a difficult time finding work at a call center. After being hired, she was trained to neutralize her accent, given a new moniker more user-friendly and culturally familiar for the consumer, and exposed to the popular culture and idioms of the US location she would be calling. After the initial excitement of her first professional job wore off, she began to feel the toll of her nighttime work schedule. She became increasingly disconnected to her daytime social world, family, and friends, and she finally felt like her daytime self went through something like a social death.[1] At this point she quit her job. Having gone directly into a call center after college, however, Bharati soon found that her only job skills, including a neutral accent and her knowledge of US geography, work processes, and people, were of no use to any other industry. Within 6 months she joined another call center.[2]

In another part of India, a woman of around the same age, a mother of two named Sujata-ben, signed a contract with a medical center to become a gestational carrier for a couple in the United States with fertility concerns. After going through the medical process of hormone administration and embryo transplantation to become impregnated, she moved to a hostel for gestational carriers in northern India. She explained in an interview midway through her pregnancy that she had already given birth to two children of her own, and during those pregnancies, she had not taken nearly as much care of herself or committed as much thought to her well-being as she was currently. She had been employed as a maid for the better part of both of her previous pregnancies, whereas now she lived apart from her husband, children, and family duties and spent her days passing the time with other women who shared her condition, alternating between affects of boredom and camaraderie, depending on the context. As a surrogate, she paid careful attention to the condition of the pregnancy, particularly her nutrition and rest. She also mentioned that she didn't have the attention of a doctor during her previous pregnancies, much less the kind of technologically mediated care she was receiving as the gestational surrogate to a couple from the

DOI: 10.4324/9781003353362-4

United States. Like the other surrogates working with this clinic, she had signed a contract that she would not receive any money other than a maintenance stipend if she did not successfully complete her pregnancy.[3]

The requisite adjustments to the mode of living and attention and care of the self that Bharati and Sujata-ben undertook in order to earn a living are indicative of vastly different yet parallel shifts in the conditions and valuation of new forms of labor in India. While call centers are thought of in the United States as a sign of outsourcing and often as a mark of a shift in industrialized economies to postmodern, flexible production, commercial surrogacy is not often considered labor in the same way. However, for both call center work and gestational surrogacy, the category of labor becomes essential for making visible the types of value-transmitting activities that subjects undergo for the benefit of those who consume them. Attending to these forms of labor also allows for the continued political project of tracking their accumulation and exploitation. What call center work and commercial surrogacy have in common is the labor of producing and transferring human vital energy directly to a consumer, through the work of affect and the intentional or dedicated use of bodily organs and processes. The work of producing vital energy through biological and affective labor is distributed unequally at the level of international exchange, as are opportunities for its consumption. In performing this labor with its transnational transfer of value, racialized and gendered bodies/subjects become the bearers of colonial legacies and neoliberal restructurings that create an opportunity to expand as well as think outside of current ways of conceptualizing labor. Examining these new forms of labor also provides an opportunity to reevaluate the role of race and gender in relation to subjectivity and humanity, forms of ownership and property, and technology as part of capitalist expansion and territorialization.

The production of a persona as an instrument to communicate attention and service in call center work and the commercial surrogate's allocation of time, attention, and care to her body and well-being as an instrument in producing a child by contract evoke an imagination of the proceeding edge of the expanding commodification of subjects and humanity, and as such, it is useful to think about how they also complicate a strictly labor-based analysis of this production. The geopolitical and structural location of this production, occurring in India but accumulated by consumers in the global North, including the middle and upper classes in hyperdeveloped spaces as well as the transnational capitalist class[4] and growing middle class in India, also invites connection to questions of use value, constraint, and autonomy raised by the history of imperial labor in India.

Affective and biological labor such as that found in call center and surrogacy work are indices of new forms of exploitation and accumulation within neoliberal globalization, but they also rearticulate a historical colonial division of labor. Affective and biological labor differ in kind from the productive labor that both liberal capitalism and Marxist critical analysis presume; in this sense, the attention to undertheorized labor like call center work, surrogacy, clinical trial participation, the organ trade, and so on, brings into relief both the longer imperial legacies of liberal capitalism and assesses the adequacy of Marxist critiques of political economy as a framework of analysis. Feminist materialist analyses of the historical differentiation of productive and reproductive labor are an invaluable resource for articulating the limits of both liberal and Marxist notions of labor, value, and political subjectivity. Yet even as these feminist materialists point to the unwaged, unrecognized reproductive, or even "maternal," labors of service, care, and nurture, they fall short of identifying how exploitation of gendered labor is also part of a system that governs through reduction and extension of "life" or what Michel Foucault elaborates as "biopower," which depends on these degraded feminized labors, even as it uses them up. While arguing that the category of reproductive labor makes visible a type of productivity that is essential yet unseen, this scholarship also provides the grounds to continue to scrutinize which kinds of exchange and subjectivity can even be represented by categories of labor. Such analyses thus lead us to ask specifically what stakes are involved in asserting that gestational surrogates and others whose productivity occurs primarily through biological and affective processes are subjects of capitalist labor power.

The affective and biological exploitation and accumulation represented together in call centers and commercial surrogacy depend as much on contemporary technologies that disaggregate and commodify discrete acts as they do on the longer colonial political economy within which human "life" (as free, autonomous, self-willing, and biologically healthy) has been supported in the First World by the labor and materials of the Third. A rereading of the undertheorized side of the dual nature of reproductive labor remains essential for understanding the co-constitution of the sexual organization of the heteropatriarchal family and the work of gendered labor both to humanize workers for continued production and to provide a source of unmarked accumulation in itself. Structures of race and gender continue to disguise the transmission of vital energy, that is, the value imparted by labor and more, between bodies and communities. In addition to creating value recognizable through exchange, the duality of this labor contributes to the sexualized humanizing project and accumulation that feminist materialist scholars locate in the heteropatriarchal family as a privileged form of life. On a more general level, it also helps characterize India's (racialized) role as a primary provider in the gendered global service economy.

Studying the accumulation of vital energy as a form of "biocapital"[5] in these processes provides a way to specify what is different and the same about this particular economy in ways that modern liberal or Marxist concepts—freedom or consent, on the one hand, or exchange and surplus value, on the other—cannot accommodate. Tracking vital energy, rather than value, as the content of what is produced and transmitted between biological and affective producers and their consumers holds on to the human vitality that Karl Marx describes as the true content of value carried by the commodity and the absolute use value of labor power to capitalist production, while maintaining the argument that what is produced by these activities exceeds what is recognizable in the commodity's exchange value. It makes plain the connection between the exhaustion of biological bodies and labors in India to extend "life" in the First World and a longer history of power relations under-pinning what may seem like an emerging form of biopower in sites like commercial surrogacy.

Material Feminism and the Dual Nature of Reproductive Labor

> The production of immediate life in all its aspects must be the core concept of a feminist theory of labor.
>
> —Maria Mies, Patriarchy and Accumulation on a World Scale

The vignette above about Bharati is taken from the portrait of a composite call center agent produced by the sociologist A. Aneesh from interviews conducted in the New Delhi industrial suburb of Gurgaon.[6] An important part of becoming a call center agent, where practical training occurs after hiring but before paid work begins, is the acquisition of fluency in the foreign culture he or she is calling, so that an agent may react appropriately and credibly to customers in their own cultural context. For example, agents must acquire the habit of showing culturally authentic emotions on the phone, such as performing empathy for a customer who relates a misfortune or keeping a smile on his or her face during the conversation. These efforts translate into the production of value for their employers in the form of increased customer trust and loyalty to the company or brand. In addition to the affective work of producing their caller personas, the time difference between India and North America means that call center agents are required to do the daily work of managing the friction created by waking up late in the afternoon when others are winding down their days and missing social engagements, religious rituals, and the other everyday interactions that constitute sociality.

The projected persona of the call center agent turns out to be more useful to the global economy than the subject that projects it as a worker. Most of the college-educated middle-class young adults employed by call centers profess their lack of interest in call center work yet are attracted by the pay and the idea that this is something they can do to earn money for a few years while they find a "real job."[7] In truth, when an agent tries to leave the call center industry, he or she often finds that the skills used in call center work are employable only in other call centers. The "real" worker, as opposed to the agent's performed persona, is revealed to be flawed in terms of market demands. The transformation of the agent into her projected caller persona requires the suppression of her real form and yet results in the enhancement of her life opportunities because it gives her access to global flows of capital and labor demands. Her primary opportunity to earn a wage is found in producing and reproducing the caller persona.

The story of Bharati's necessary alienation from social relations and her social world, resulting from the temporal and cultural isolation of call center work from other industries and work schedules, combined with her access to a job only through the work of affect that reproduces an alternate subject, engages the concerns of feminist analyses of labor. It also raises questions about the specific content of the call center agent's labor, which includes supporting a projected persona who occupies an alien world that the agent must learn and then inhabit through fantasy. Agents also do the work of managing the emotional reactions, expectations, and communication between depersonalized entities like brands or corporations and individual people, reassuring them of their worth and existence as human beings. The blurring of the line between the subject and the work performed lends call center work to analysis as reproductive and gendered labor, which is distinguished by tasks and contexts in which it is difficult to distinguish the line between the body and subject of the worker and the work performed. Such tasks and work contexts point to the complexities of assuming autonomy when work involves affective and biological participation and alienation, and gestures to the vast range of activities that fall into the "production of immediate life" that Maria Mies forefronts as the necessary core concept of a feminist theory of labor in the epigraph above.

The second vignette, excerpted from ethnographic observation and interviews conducted in 2008, takes place at a residence hostel in a small city in the Indian province of Gujarat, where women who are in different stages of pregnancy and postdelivery as contracted gestational surrogates live for 9 months to a year while working with the Manushi fertility clinic.[8] The context of surrogacy varies from clinic to clinic in India, as there are only elective national guidelines for commercial assisted reproductive technology practice, but most clinics mandate or heavily encourage surrogates to live in designated hostels. Many, including Manushi, only accept married women who have borne at least one child in order to prove the viability of their uteruses and to work against their possible attachment to the fetus/infant. The latter requirement has also been written into draft legislation.[9] Sujata-ben's narrative describes self-care, concern, caution, and attention, which exemplify some of the affective labor and commodities produced by a surrogate while pregnant. These and the breast-feeding and nurturing of the newborn she may be asked to provide generate health and therefore yield future life opportunities for both the infant and its parents.

As a paid service, commercial surrogacy is imagined in the context of the clinic as the contractual usage of a woman's otherwise unused uterus as a space in which to gestate a fetus that is understood as someone else's property and progeny. On the one hand, surrogacy is a contracted agreement of payment for the gestation of a fetus created through in vitro fertilization and the delivery of an infant. However, the custodianship and intentional continued gestation of the fetus lend themselves in practice and in proposed legislation to the need to protect consumers by mandating that a woman submit herself to technologies and routine surveillance that is meant to protect the well-being of the fetus, sometimes more than that of the surrogate herself.

The surrogacy fee, which is highly attractive for surrogates but much lower than what commissioning parents would pay in their home countries, reflects a "lower cost of living" in their different spheres of life. The fee is also attractive to India's urban transnational capitalist class who share a similar earning differential with surrogates. Surrogates describe the unparalleled earning opportunity surrogacy represents by providing a sum that could actually change their material circumstances. Due to their lower incomes, surrogates often do without many necessities that commissioning parents would not do without, including basic health insurance, medical privacy, reliable electricity, clean and reliable water, a permanent home/residence, the ability to seek and find another job when one is lost, access to a variety of foods or the ability to grow them (requiring land and water), and so on. This disparity of conditions and access to resources is not accurately reflected in the argument that Indian surrogates' fees are low because of the lower cost of living of the women who become surrogates. Transnational surrogates in India hired by distant commissioning parents provide an opportunity for commissioning couples to continue to live at home, maintain their paid work, and build their careers in lieu of childbearing, even as surrogates themselves relocate and give up their other work to provide this opportunity.

As emerging case law in a number of countries allowing transnational commercial surrogacy has begun to illustrate, the social relations and understandings of kinship outside the medical and legal definitions of the surrogacy contract are not as simple as represented in the agreement of 9 months of gestation and childbirth in exchange for a set fee. In fact, surrogates themselves insist on the continuing obligation and duty commissioning parents should feel toward them and their families beyond the terms and time limit of the contract, arguing that the act of giving a child to a wanting couple is incommensurable with any fee. Even in the face of evidence that commissioning parents rarely keep up correspondence or support of a woman and her family after the surrogacy contract has ended, many describe the expectation that this should be so, given the relative power and resources of commissioning parents and the nature of what surrogates have given them in bearing their child.[10] The call of such a duty or responsibility doesn't transmit between the surrogate and the commissioning parent because of the organizing rubrics of the liberal, individual subject and the contract-based relationship that describes the responsibility of each party in terms of fee and service rendered.[11] These expectations also point to a disagreement about the value of surrogacy as labor and about its content, which exceed what can be understood in terms of value and the autonomous, liberal individual subject.

An understanding of how the production of immediate life through affect and biology on one side of the world can serve to support life elsewhere is aided by an examination of the dual nature of the type of labor that is often referred to as "reproductive." Marx's formulation from volume 1 of Capital defines reproductive labor against productive labor. If productive labor is understood as the investment of (socially averaged) labor time into an object for exchange, then reproductive labor is the energy put into making sure the person doing productive labor was able to return to work each day. It re-creates or replenishes the labor power of the person who works outside the home in the public sphere by providing support to the biological reproduction of the worker's body and strength, as well as a replacement worker in the form of child rearing. In the form of care, love, and nurture, it also reassures the worker of his humanity, allowing him to continue to participate in his own commodification as labor.

Contemporary feminists have extended this analysis by redefining such labor as productive in itself, producing immediate life and not just supporting the masculine worker who earned the means to immediate subsistence.[12] As a result of this history of the feminization of work that reproduces life, work that often involves a service rather than a physical object as its commodity, service and care also remain undervalued in public labor markets. Service, care, and attention work are considered unskilled because they originated in a gendered division of labor that did not require the identification of skills to secure a contract, as this was covered in contracts of marriage and servitude.[13] At the same time, a growing percentage of jobs, particularly those performed by people marginalized in a given society or within the international division of labor, are these very jobs of care and service.

Affective and biological labors differ in kind from the productive labor that Marx presumes and analyzes in volume 1 of Capital; that is, the labor of the worker who sews a coat or makes a chair meant for exchange is different than the call center worker or the surrogate, in that the latter workers engage in both productive and reproductive labors. Activities of service, care, and nurture engage the biological use of their bodies and lives as well as labor, and the requirements of such work intrude on the laboring subject in ways that radically compromise any sense of "autonomy" or "separation of spheres" presumed by both liberal and Marxist discussions of workers within western societies. Biotechnology together with globalization (and its colonial past) is the condition that makes the selling or renting of one's biological function and parts possible, a process that is qualitatively different than the commodification of the labor that the biological body performs.

Both commercial surrogacy and call center work produce recognizable commodities in exchange for a monetary sum (stipend/fee and wage, respectively). They also produce a number of other use values including feelings or affects, forms of sociality and humanity, and the valorization of those forms among their consumers. Occurring in the domestic/nonpublic realm and producing commodities that do not line up with a physical model, elements of domestic work have often not been visible as productive or even as labor to mainstream political economic labor analysis, nor to philosophies of labor that privilege a liberal autonomous individual as the subject of capitalist labor. As a result, domestic work and reproductive work in general, as well as the subject who performs them, get represented, at least in part, as nonvalue.[14] To address this problem, Leopoldina Fortunati has identified a dual nature within capital's appropriation of labor power, a dualism that is within labor power itself. Reproductive work, a category in which domestic work is a large component, has a dual nature under capitalism because it represents itself and its subject/bearer as nonvalue, yet it simultaneously functions to siphon the value it produces into capital through the ability of the "productive" worker to return to work each day.[15] Fortunati's understanding of reproduction as inherent but unmarked in the value of labor power is a very different approach to that of earlier feminist models of domestic work as either productive labor deserving of a wage or as reproductive labor coerced by patriarchy. Approaching affective labor in this way allows us to see its essential role of compensating and rehumanizing the worker as more than a commodity, "creating the illusion that he is an individual with unique characteristics and a real personality."[16]

The material predication of the subject of capitalist labor as "labor power" is based on the idea that what makes us useful to capital as embodied subjects is the surplus of vital energy we can commit to activity beyond what we need to sustain life and productivity of the individual and its extension into a replacement worker (in the form of the worker's child). Commercial surrogacy, because of its social location in mothering labor and the cultural-economic weight of the household/family economic unit that comes with that location, together with its imbrication with the bodies of producer and consumer, complicates the surrogate as a capitalist worker-subject. Feminist theory in different areas has shown that the subject of labor power relies on a host of supports that originate in the vital energy of others, supports that do not appear to be labor or behave like it. These include the historical structure of the Protestant heteropatriarchal household with its wives, children, and servants, as well as through colonization, indenture, and slavery, as these have obscured subjects of value-producing labor in support of the subject predicated by labor power in the capitalist market.

Janet Jakobsen argues that "the autonomous individual is not just any particular human being but a particular way to understand and inhabit human being—a subjectivity in which the individual understands himself to be free when he acts without the assistance of others,"[17] an understanding of autonomy that obscures the support labor of those upon whom this autonomy depends. For this reason, Jakobsen argues that sexual relations within the Protestant heteropatriarchal family are relations of production that produce both the autonomous individual and this particular variety of human subject.[18] Indian gestational surrogacy falls into this sexual mode of production as the privatized labor of reproduction and childbirth. It is also crucial to note that when surrogates insist that their role exceeds that of gestational carrier, they are challenging the individuality, freedom, and private quality of this mode of production,[19] as well as revealing the work that goes into supporting it through contracts, legislation, and assumed norms of sociality and kinship.

Housewifization, colonization, and the global elaboration of these and other legacies in "flexibilization"[20] are part of the history that leads to the present-day understanding of commercial surrogacy. Bringing gendered labor, with its ties to property and patriarchy, under the umbrella of labor remains the most effective way to gain protections for a variety of subjects. For example, feminists in India have historically conducted efforts and continue to push the government toward a future that opens up opportunities for women with regard to reproductive technologies and equality of representation and access to rights over property, progeny, labor, and their own bodies.[21] In this context, organizations like Sama: Resource Group for Women and Health in New Delhi, a national research and advocacy group, have introduced the issue of transnational surrogacy. Sociologist Amrita Pande suggests that the model of labor organization and demands for labor protections is the immediate concern from the vantage of the needs of women working as surrogates, despite the obstacles to surrogates' realization of a worker's consciousness.[22] However, the model of "ownership" of the body as a solution to the problem of identifying the value of gendered bodily labor does not address the problem of the devaluation of women's bodies, particularly the maternal body under patriarchal property-based systems where "the bodies are just the space in which the genetic material matures into babies," and if the body is believed to contain the property of someone else, owning her body is not enough to ensure the maternal subject's civil liberties.[23]

The woman acting as a gestational surrogate, much like the colonized laborer, the housewife, and the worker outside of labor protections, is partially a subject of labor who is "free" to sell labor to buyers but is also occluded as a subject in the service of what Mies and Fortunati have identified as ongoing primitive accumulation. Defined as housewives rather than workers, women become the ideal labor force, because the full use value and productivity of their work is obscured, since it does not appear or circulate as "free wage labor."[24] Lacking definition as true income-generating activities, intentional actions that transmit life-supporting energy and the reaffirmation of humanness can create value through commodities but also directly support life in other bodies, communities, and locations.

Technology has played an important role in separating the pregnant body as a productive machine from the subject, freeing the work of gestation and nurture to circulate as commodities. However, examination of the history of slavery and indenture in India itself and as part of British colonial labor allocation in the colonies adds an additional and important layer for considering the content of labor that is understood to be produced by a free, liberal subject, a tension that complements the analysis of the dual nature of reproductive labor, where part of what is produced necessarily remains outside the reach of recognizing the subject of such work as a subject of labor.

Legacies of Imperial Labor

> The social inequalities of our time are a legacy of this definition of "the human" and subsequent discourses that have placed particular subjects, practices, and geographies at a distance from "the human."
>
> —Lisa Lowe, "The Intimacies of Four Continents"

As the quotation from Lisa Lowe above asserts, the emergence of humanism as a liberal philosophy of the subject, organized through a distinction of freedom from conditions of unfreedom, was co-constituted by the formation of colonial racial categorizations and an international division of labor as they arose together following the abolition of the slave trade within the British Empire in 1807.[25] Madhavi Kale's study of the recruitment and resettlement of bonded or indentured laborers from India to the Caribbean argues that empire was the invisible pretext for the constitution of labor as an identity and as a category of analysis in historiography.[26] The distinction between enslaved and free labor that became a concern as part of the abolitionist movement functioned to generate a category of mobile workers that complemented an imperial labor reallocation strategy connecting imperial subjects all over the world as "labor" while elaborating their hierarchical relationship and separation through emerging categories of race and gender attached to their labor. In turn, the nature of freedom and free labor became invested with assumptions about gender, race, and class,[27] as they were also embroiled in the instrumental distinction between free labor and slavery that justified the practice of indenture. This instrumentality wrote over the coercive nature of indenture since it was described as contractual by mutual consent and understanding, even in the face of evidence of the lack of understanding or choice on the part of those signing themselves into indenture. Women were recruited under the same contractual conditions as men, though for the purpose of providing the reproductive labor that made male workers viable, a practice and problem that Kale asserts is embedded in the material origins of the category of free labor as an instrument in imperial labor real-location. This reallocation was in effect the superimposition of a constructed dichotomy of slavery and free labor on the proliferation of less-than-free labor and conditions as part of empire building, whereby "the post-abolitionist fiction of equal status and equal protection for all imperial subjects regardless of race or nation could be maintained by erasing women as political agents," what Lowe calls a "modern racial governmentality."[28] Like the fiction of noncoercion underpinning Indian indenture, in the larger colonial context of the British Empire, a number of gendered, sexual, and reproductive relations existed under the umbrella of "consensual" that did not even figure as labor.[29] Abstract notions of "consent," "freedom," "choice," and "contract" have been produced and unequally distributed by modern liberalism, have been affirmed selectively for some through the disavowal of colonized and enslaved labor,[30] and continue to write over contemporary conditions of force under other names.[31]

These histories, together with the history of the category of free labor itself, mandate attention be paid not only to the particular nature of the work being performed under contract in emerging affective and biological production, but also to the particular forms of dependency in operation, as such contractual arrangements may contain incomplete or absent information and consent, and therefore incomplete autonomy, despite being arranged through a freely entered contractual agreement.

For example, the contemporary status of women who take up gestational surrogacy is particular in a number of ways. It is constructed through Indian law, particularly through legal relations that accord little power to the surrogate. The draft Assisted Reproductive Technologies Bill considered by India's Parliament in several redrafts between 2010 and 2016 was largely a free-market-promoting document that provides only basic protections to surrogates as under-resourced Indian citizens. Therefore the practice of commercial surrogacy was subject only to national guidelines that are not enforceable. The status of women once they enter into a surrogacy agreement is also defined through the translation of human gestation into paid labor; they may receive trimesterly stipends as they proceed through pregnancy, and after delivering the infant, they receive their fees. This means that once she becomes pregnant, the surrogate must complete the pregnancy to receive payment, and as it stands in the draft bill, the surrogate would not have a say in decisions about embryo reduction or abortion. There is currently no legal guarantee of medical treatment for complications arising after the delivery, and there is no formal procedure to follow should anything untoward happen to the woman while pregnant. Her legal status as a particular kind of worker whose body has been engaged through a contract to perform self-care and nurture with the aim of a healthy pregnancy and delivery does not account for the frequent separation enforced between surrogates and their nuclear and extended families and communities in the interest of the clinic and commissioning parents, nor does it account for any effects of her own separation from the child she bears. There is no socially recognizable or defensible relationship between the surrogate's social world and that of the infant she carries other than the contract, even in the proposed legislation. This separation is figured as natural and commonsensical within the discourses of biological parenthood and property, where intention and gametes on the part of commissioning parents give them ownership of the embryo, fetus, and infant and as such is endorsed by the clinic through its contract with the surrogate. The surrogate has no claim on the developing fetus and is in fact positioned in the current guidelines and proposed legislation as a potential threat to it. Current contracts may also forbid the surrogate from engaging in sexual intercourse with her husband and may effectively mandate residence in surrogate hostels to facilitate surveillance.

These conditions raise questions that escape the reach of even the well-meaning and necessary efforts to gain labor protections for women working as surrogates in India. They engage an imperial history of instrumentalizing consent, freedom and choice, alienation, and sexual and reproductive relations made invisible as labor while their subjects disappear from the identity category of labor through their gendering and the gendering of their work. While all biological life represents a site of speculation and potential biological production and accumulation, the legacies of imperialism continue to affect the hyperavailability of racialized and gendered bodies.[32] The concerns raised by the legacies of colonial labor in India come to bear upon the social alienation and constraint of choice among workers in the call center industry and other forms of gendered industrial labor, as these value-producing activities straddle the line of visible and invisible labor, autonomy, and coercion, while engaging interior levels of the subject, self, and personality in their performance.

Biology, Autonomy, and Liberal Humanism

> [The way we understand agency and the political] has a range of consequences and effects that concern the constitution of the subject . . . [including] the incommensurability of liberal notions of will and autonomy as standards for evaluating subaltern behavior.
>
> —Saidiya Hartman, Scenes of Subjection

As Sujata-ben's story suggests, the way surrogates compare previous pregnancies to contracted pregnancy through surrogacy, specifically the different orientation to the process and to their bodies, raises the questions of what affective labor is invested into gestation and what resultant commodities are produced by the surrogate's self-care while pregnant. Many women are asked to provide 2 days of breast-feeding after delivery to give the infant immunity-building colostrum, but occasionally this period is extended for 1 or 2 months for infants whose parents are delayed in their arrival. In addition to expanding the range of subject positions one can inhabit as "mother" both as capitalist laborer and as excessive to capitalist production, assisted reproductive technologies also create future opportunities for less-wealthy women to step into devalued care labor markets and for more wealthy women to outsource the work of childbearing and child rearing in order to expand their own ability to pursue full-time careers through their reproductive years, a process that, in the context of transnational adoption, Ann Anagnost calls "just-in-time" reproduction.[33]

Race and gender have historically operated and continue to operate to make some bodies more economically useful as biological entities than as the subjects of labor power. In the context of commercial gestational surrogacy in India, part of the work being done by the distinction between "gestational carrier" and "commissioning parent" in the clinical context is distinguishing a separation between the physical aspects of human reproduction and the social/sexual/affective aspects. Much of the work of the clinic staff is invested in preventing the attachment of emotional meaning to relationships between surrogates and commissioning parents and between the surrogate and the fetus she carries. As a sign within the discourse of genetic essentialism, the gene distinguishes the provider of the service and reproductive space of gestation from the creative "author" of the child—the "biological parents." Patriarchy—as assumed and affirmed through the state and supporting legal apparatuses, including paternity and property protections at the national level that are built into documents like the surrogacy contract itself—identifies the commissioning parents as the intentional authors of a future child protected as property, though necessarily under the custodianship of the surrogate for the period of gestation.

Scientific knowledge and practices have played a role in erasing bodies from reproduction in surrogacy. For example, in the context of commercial surrogacy, genetic discourse dictates the property-bearing and contract-empowered status of the commissioning parents as the intentional, authorial producers of a child; the embryologist and obgyn form a technical team that performs the high-value work of engineering the surrogacy, leaving the surrogate positioned as performing the passive, merely reproductive and non-authorial work of gestation. How is a fetus produced? In vitro fertilization involves skills, knowledge, and instruments that require specialized training and education, as does the implantation of an embryo in concert with the administration of hormones to prepare a surrogate's body to become pregnant with the implanted embryo. The surrogate continues the process through to its completion, and her body uses its complex biological and hormonal mechanisms to bring the fetus to term, mechanisms that are influenced by her activities during gestation (nutrition, stress level, exposure to mutagenic substances, physical activity, health, or illness, among others).

As the quotation from Saidiya Hartman above argues, attention to different subject formations and potential subalterneity marks the need for caution in approaching agency and political activity, particularly as these are often tied up in property relations. The way these activities are read as being labor or not, and as being specialized or not, is heavily influenced by the assumption that the end product is a form of contract-protected property belonging to the originators of intention and DNA. However, as one representative genetic biologist explains, "First, DNA is not self-reproducing, second, it makes nothing, and third, organisms are not determined by it."[34] While "women's experience confounds the dichotomy of manual/mental labor,"[35] we can recognize that there have been important historical precedents for the structures of race, gender, patriarchy, and imperialism in the commercialization of this labor that have simultaneously erased much of its content. The wealthy have always hired out this labor along class, race, gender, and national differentials, and the boundaries between women's bodies and society, the social, and the public have always been considered porous in different contexts. However, the distribution of wealth in the world has changed so that gendered labor, still performed by individuals marked hierarchically as having low social status, has to travel farther to reach them. Also, a shift in how privacy and property are being defined is part of the growth of the service sector.

The example of gestational surrogacy is an obvious illustration of how intimate expression, requiring the production of genuine feelings, can be completely alienated from the producer. The time surrogates spend away from their families and communities, which many surrogates describe as the most taxing element of their work, and away from the social and biological activities that produce their own immediate life and life world is invested into the lives of consumers and their environment in immediately observable ways.[36] The rapid growth of commercialized affect and biological economies raises questions about how their growth impacts our activities outside the realm of exchange. For example, in a system mediated by private property, where sensuality becomes colonized by the sense of "having," does caring for children in support of another household or other microeconomy for artificially low compensation undervalue the labor you do in your own home?[37] Does it devalue the effects associated with love?[38] Can it create a surplus of commodified love in the world that cheapens the affective content of the life of the worker who still cannot afford to consume it herself?[39] At the same time that these questions acknowledge the infinite set of needs that must be denied to devalued subjects/workers as a condition of rendering their bodies and life energies "surplus" and available for export, we must also continually raise the imperial history of labor that refuses the classification of free labor—that is humanity itself—to the imperial subjects of capital. In other words, not all labor is visible as such, and capitalist value (among other things) is created by both proper subjects as well as those who do not always appear as (liberal) subjects. To accurately follow value's production and accumulation therefore requires attention to the availability of autonomy in a given production setting.

Conclusion

When gestational surrogates enter into contracts with commissioning parents in the United States or call center workers expend affective effort to manage the emotions of US customers, these surrogates and call center workers enter into layers of other historical contexts that prefigure them in important ways. For example, in transmitting vital energy to US residents, they enter into a history of US capitalist accumulation in relation to conquest, racial slavery, and immigration, where the reproductive labor of working-class women of color continues to support the value of whiteness and class privilege that does not include them. The quality of this accumulation, historically invested into the white US middle class, is important and serves an instrumental purpose not unlike the freeing of Indian workers to become bonded labor in the Caribbean under the British Empire.

In addition to investing unquantified value into these families and households, the devaluing of racialized and gendered service work has perpetuated a discourse of white middle- and upper-middle-class families as needing more care than working-class families and families of color.[40] This has led to a naturalized lifestyle difference that continues to validate more care and affective resources in some homes, whereas in others these are what Rosemary Hennessey calls "outlawed necessities."[41] Mies observes a similar result in the reduced material ability of women in the global South to realize an idealized femininity defined against the "civilized" modern woman.[42] This gap creates the very conditions of dehumanization under which she must work more and more to lower the cost of production of what others can buy (rather than what she needs) to support the material feasibility of the "producer-housewife" in the global North.[43]

As indicated by the analysis of the dual nature of reproductive labor, affective and biological labor can serve not just to reproduce capital, property, and the conditions under which capital and property continue to exist, but also can contribute to the unquantifiable ability of consuming classes to thrive in a way that presents a continuation and increase of present opportunities into an unforeseeable future, to make the consumer feel "more human," and to continue to disenfranchise the humanity of those whose unrecognized productivity allows for this investment. The question of what is produced through gestational surrogacy includes the way that futurity is imagined through the biological child and technologically informed notions of kinship that lead us back to property, rights, and biopower as unstable future political propositions.

Notes

I'd like to thank Melinda Cooper and Terry Woronov for careful readings of early drafts of this piece in their role as editors and for comments that greatly strengthened its arguments. A writing group with Sora Han, Rashad Shabazz, and Pascha Bueno-Hansen offered comments on a very early draft. Advice from Neda Atanasoski and Julietta Hua was instrumental in helping conceptualize the essay's form and structure, and their editorial comments were extremely valuable. I am also grateful to Lisa Lowe, Nathan Camp, Roshanak Kheshti, and Meg Wesling for their insightful and generative feedback.

1 A. Aneesh. (2007). "Specters of Global Communication," *Frakcija*, 43–44: 26–33.
2 Ibid.
3 Excerpted from ethnographic interviews conducted by author, Gujarat, India, January–February 2008.
4 A. Aneesh. (2006). *Virtual Migration: The Programming of Globalization* (Durham, NC: Duke University Press), 18.
5 Sarah Franklin. (2001). "Ethical Biocapital: New Strategies of Cell Culture," in *Remaking Life and Death*, Sarah Franklin and Margaret Lock, eds. (Santa Fe, NM: School of American Research Press); Kaushik Sunder Rajan. (2006). *Biocapital: The Constitution of Postgenomic Life* (Durham, NC: Duke University Press). Sarah Franklin and Kaushik Sunder Rajan have used the concept of biocapital to describe the rise of biological information as commodities and capital. I expand this formulation of biocapital to examine the commodification of body parts and the vitality of biological and affective energies and services. This more inclusive use of the concept of biocapital provides a way to understand, within a capitalist framework and from a feminist perspective, how surrogacy and the work of care and attention can act as forms of productive labor through the investment of human vital energy directly into another person, family, and society to support their continued life.
6 Aneesh, "Specters."
7 Ben Addelman et al., dirs. (2006). "Bombay Calling," https://en.wikipedia.org/wiki/Bombay_Calling.
8 The clinic's name has been changed.
9 The draft Assisted Reproductive Technologies Bill. (2010). http://icmr.nic.in/guide/ART%20REGULATION%20Draft%20Bill1.pdf, Accessed April 26, 2012.
10 Kalindi Vora. (2010). "Medicine, Markets and the Pregnant Body: Indian Commercial Surrogacy and Reproductive Labor in a Transnational Frame," *Scholar and Feminist Online*, 9(1–2), http://barnard.edu/sfonline/reprotech/vora_01.htm.
11 Surrogates have little power to pursue breach of contract by commissioning parents or the clinic, and anecdotal evidence from news reports and the documentary film Made in India suggest that surrogates often do not receive the full fee they have been promised. Rebecca Haimowitz and Vaishali Sinha, dirs.

(2010). *Made in India: A Film about Surrogacy*. New York: Chicken and Egg Pictures.

12 Queer theorists in particular have challenged the idea of reproductivity by troubling the meaning of care work as simply reproducing what was already there, arguing instead that new forms of life and family life are produced that do not line up with the imperatives of the heteropatriarchal household economy. See Ann Cvetkovich (2003). *An Archive of Feelings: Trauma, Sexuality, and Lesbian Public Cultures* (Durham, NC: Duke University Press); José Esteban Muñoz. (2020). *The Sense of Brown: Ethnicity, Affect, and Performance* (Durham, NC: Duke University Press).

13 Maria Mies. (1986). *Patriarchy and Accumulation on a World Scale: Women in the International Division of Labour* (London: Third World Books).

14 Leopoldina Fortunati. (1989). *The Arcane of Reproduction: Housework, Prostitution, Labor and Capital*, trans. Hilary Creek, ed. Jim Fleming (New York: Autonomedia), 9–13.

15 Ibid., 9–10.

16 Ibid., 110.

17 Janet Jakobsen. (2012). "Perverse Justice," *GLQ: A Journal of Lesbian and Gay Studies*, 18(1): 25.

18 Ibid.

19 See Vora. (2010). "Medicine, Markets."

20 The feminization of domestic labor through what Maria Mies calls "housewifization," a process that extended from the late Middle Ages through the Enlightenment in Europe and coincided with the witch pogroms, also naturalized women's work within the household so that it could be treated in the same way as natural resources and colonial labor—as a free good to be exploited in a one-way relationship. Identifying the work of the housewife as organized for ongoing primitive accumulation, Mies claims that it continues to be the secret of modern capitalist expansion (1986). Claudia von Werlhof argues that the process of breaking up trade unions and "flexibilizing" labor locates many male workers outside the protection of labor laws, which positions their labor much like that of women's domestic labor. Claudia von Werlhof. (1988). "The Proletarian Is Dead: Long Live the Housewife?," in *Women: The Last Colony*, Maria Mies, Veronika Bennholdt-Thomsen and Claudia von Werlhof, eds. (London: Zed Books), 254–264.

21 See Rajeswari Sundar Rajan, *The Scandal of the State: Women, Law, and Citizenship in Postcolonial India* (Durham, NC: Duke University Press, 2003).

22 Amrita Pande. (2010). "Commercial Surrogacy in India: Manufacturing a Perfect Mother-Worker," *Feminist Studies*, 35(4): 969–992.

23 Barbara Katz Rothman. (2000). *Recreating Motherhood* (New Brunswick, NJ: Rutgers University Press).

24 Fortunati, *The Arcane of Reproduction*, 116.

25 Ibid.

26 Madhavi Kale, *Fragments of Empire: Capital, Slavery, and Indian Indentured Labor in the British Caribbean* (Philadelphia, PA: University of Pennsylvania Press, 1998), 4.

27 Ibid., 7.

28 Lisa Lowe. (2015). *Intimacies of Four Continents* (Durham: Duke University Press), 174, 194.

29 Ibid., 195.

30 Ibid.

31 In his study of human indenture and slavery in India, Lakshmidhar Mishra defines forced labor as that which "deprives a person of the choice of alternative of work/avocation, compels him to adopt one particular course of action which is usually abhorrent to him." Lakshmidhar Mishra. (2011). *Human Bondage: Tracing Its Roots in India* (New Delhi: Sage Publications), 43.

32 Lawrence Cohen calls the intersection of poverty and advances in biotechnology to yield the bodies and body parts of impoverished Indian kidney sellers over others' bioavailability, a term also describing the emergence of women in working and lower middle- class India as gestational surrogates. Lawrence Cohen. (2005). "Operability, Bioavailability, and Exception," in *Global Assemblages: Technology, Politics, and Ethics and Anthropological Problems*, Aihwa Ong and Stephen J. Collier, eds. (Malden, MA: Blackwell Publishing), 79–90.

33 Ann Anagnost. (2000). "Scenes of Misrecognition: Maternal Citizenship in the Age of Transnational Adoption," *Positions*, 8(2): 389–421.

34 Richard C. Lewontin. (1992). "The Dream of the Human Genome," *New York Review of Books*, May 28, cited in Donna Haraway. (1997). *ModestWitness@Second_Millennium.Female-Man_Meets_OncoMouse: Feminism and Technoscience* (New York: Routledge), 145.

35 Nancy C.M. Hartsock. (1983). "The Feminist Standpoint: Developing the Ground for a Specifically Feminist Historical Materialism," in *Discovering Reality*, Sandra Harding and Merrill B. Hintikka, eds. (Dordrecht: D. Reidel), 283–310, 299, cited in Emily Martin. (2001). *The Woman in the Body: A Cultural Analysis of Reproduction* (Boston: Beacon Press), 199.

36 Pande, "Commercial Surrogacy in India"; Vora, "Medicine, Markets."

37 Karl Marx and Friedrich Engels. (1978). "The Economic and Philosophical Manuscripts of 1844," in *The Marx-Engels Reader*, Robert C. Tucker, ed., 2nd edition. (New York: Norton), 87.

38 Pande, "Commercial Surrogacy in India"; Vora, "Medicine, Markets."

39 As Marx imagines it, the more things there are in the world, the more the vitality of the producer is scattered and the less integrity the worker has as a human. Marx and Engels, "Economic and Philosophical Manuscripts," 71.

40 See, for example, Jennifer Morgan. (2004). *Laboring Women: Reproduction and Gender in New World Slavery* (Philadelphia, PA: University of Pennsylvania Press).

41 Rosemary Hennessey. (2000). *Profit and Pleasure: Sexual Identities in Late Capitalism* (New York: Routledge).

42 Mies, *Patriarchy*, 120.

43 Ibid., 95, 118–120.

5

RE-IMAGINING REPRODUCTION

Unsettling Metaphors in the History of Imperial Science and Commercial Surrogacy in India

The rapid escalation of global access to in vivo services is enabled by the low-resourced Indian citizens who serve as surrogates (Vora 2012, 2013). Since 2004, India emerged as a premiere location for fertility tourism and ART services. However, this availability of resources for a potential market in fertility travel and surrogacy does not completely answer the question raised by Amrita Pande: Why, with India's historical antinatalism and low rates of medicalization of reproduction, is there a "labor market" for surrogates based on pronatal technologies (2014, 33). The designation of Indian labor as reproductive and service-oriented in the global economy intersects with the availability of medically- and technically trained middle-class professionals whose education was supported by programs intended to boost the newly independent Indian nation through training in applied science and technology (Francis 2001; Prashad 2007, 65). This congruence allowed Indian physicians and medical technicians to meet what came to be an increasing global demand for ARTs and surrogacy—costly and highly regulated practices highly in many high-resourced capitalist countries. Thus, in addition to low-resourced citizens, the transnational market is enabled by a population of well-trained medical professionals that arose in part because of socialized education and a national focus on science and technology education, as well as the demand in other countries for immigrant doctors, which encouraged students in India to pursue medicine as part of aspirations to migrate.

At the same time, the availability of such professionals has a much longer history than that of the recent neoliberal demand for medical technologies and professional services from the global south. India's economic development as a provider of fertility services in the global economy has historical roots in India's relationship to western medicine and in the international division of labor in British colonial practices, part of the development of global outsourcing to India. Bringing these intertwined historical relationships and contemporary disparities in medical and legal protections to bear upon reflections on recent innovations in artificial uterine environments, I suggest that the metaphors we use to structure our understanding of bodies

DOI: 10.4324/9781003353362-5

and body parts impact how we imagine appropriate roles for people and their bodies in ways that are still deeply entangled with imperial histories of science. The techno-fantasy of the isolated womb is part of the originating conditions for the structure and discourse of Indian surrogacy as "wombs for rent." The notion of the disembodied uterus that has arisen in scientific and medical practice allows for the logic of the "gestational carrier" as a functional role in assisted reproductive technologies (ART) practices. The logic of the "gestational carrier" also diminishes possible social connection and minimizes a sense of responsibility for the surrogates' life and social world apart from the time period covered by the surrogacy contract. Given these ongoing histories and metaphors, it is important to consider the unequal positions of participants in transnational fertility exchanges when evaluating recent articulations of the relationship between governance, medicine, and transnational ART markets in the debates about draft ART legislation in India. I draw upon my own and others' ethnographic research on surrogacy to address current ART practices in the context of outsourcing, which has inherited a legacy built on long held notions of feminine passivity, invisible feminized labor and the globalized gendered division of labor.

Intersecting Histories in Fertility Travel to India

The role of medicine as a discipline, and as a set of biological technologies and modes of intervention in ARTs practice is complex and multifaceted, and is as engaged with health and well-being as it is with managing bodies as resources and in disciplining social relations. In Indian transnational surrogacy practice, histories of medicine as a technique of extracting resources from human bodies and disciplining subjects intersect with legacies of British colonialism in India, where the historical role of western medicine was as tool of colonial subjectification and the British civilizing mission. This in turn helps to explain how medicine, material inequality between global populations, and the technologies of assisted reproduction come together to position low-earning women in India as instruments for the reproduction of other populations, a necessary component in fertility travel to India.

As political, economic and cultural structures have been re-organized through the stages of British colonial rule, independence and later neoliberalization in India, the relationship between western medicine, power, and the body has been cast and recast. The body and discourse about the body have historically been a site of colonization, conquest, and contestations of power in Indian history (Arnold 1988, 1993). The colonial project was an experiment in creating new types of governable subjects that both were and were not part of the same organism as British modernity. For the project of governing India as a colony, medicine and associated disciplines of bodily care were part of an experiment in creating new types of governable subjects from those under British rule at home (Prakash 1999, 127). As a result, "values of science thus played a crucial role in creating the space to displace the hegemony of the colonial mission, even while it also enabled biomedicine to justify its differentiated technologies of interventions over native and European bodies" (Towghi and Vora 2014, 11).

This legacy prefigures the way that commissioning parents, surrogates, and doctors come into relationships with one another. When commissioning parents travel to India and engage with ART clinics and Indian surrogates, they connect Indian histories with other geographically specific historical legacies, such as class relations and histories of servitude, in these sending countries. Globalization and its division of labor mapped the work of social and material reproduction onto the decolonizing global South, creating a system that evacuated resources, labor, and value from those spaces to invest it into the global North, much as the former colonial metropoles have benefitted from a similar exploitation of what world systems theory named "the peripheries" (Wallerstein 1976). Gestational surrogacy is often referred to as a new iteration of outsourcing (Hochschild 2012; Winddance-Twine 2011). The process and geography of outsourcing, where cost-effectiveness mandates locating a labor process where it is "cheapest," without concern for how that labor has been made to be cheap, genders the labor of reproduction so that some work becomes that of merely reproducing life and culture, whereas other work is deemed creative, innovative, and productive in itself (Vora 2015).

Imperial legacies undergirding contemporary practices of outsourcing also mean that we must pay attention to how we understand the politics of reproduction and labor in emerging forms of biological production and reproduction in general, but particularly in a setting like fertility travel for surrogacy, where surrogates are legally positioned as service providers versus commissioning parents, who have property rights and the rule of law to protect their access to the surrogate's services while she is pregnant. The vast gap in resources between producers and consumers in the transnational surrogacy clinic engages histories of power and difference established in India's colonial history. A historical relation of power and exploitation is evident between the Indian middle class, here represented primarily by the doctors running the clinic and by elite Indian commissioning parents, and the rural, less educated and less connected lower-class women who act as gestational surrogates. The relationship between foreign governance, Indian elites, and the rural majority population of India tracked in the work of subaltern historiographies is evident in the ART clinic, but with the added dimension of the privatization and transnational commerce entailed with the neoliberalization of India and arguably, Indian subjects.[1]

Imagining the Gendered Reproductive Body Within the Market for Fertility Services

Fertility travel to India for the purpose of surrogacy arrangements with Indian women thus points to some of the continuities and contradictions inherent in the evolution of relations between foreign economic demands, projects of the Indian elite and middle-class, and low-income rurally based Indians that have precedent in the colonial period. Here, medicine shifts from a technique of caring for the body to one of producing bodies as the instruments of service work, where the body of the surrogate is rendered available as part of an experimental economy of gestation as a service, provided by the surrogate as entrepreneur, all of which is enabled in part by the continuing relationship between medicine and the colonization of bodies in India.

The mechanical imagination of the body, an elaboration of Cartesian mind-body dualism, has nurtured a worldview in which machines can actually function as human replacements, or surrogates, at least physically if not entirely in terms of artificial intelligence. The informatization of genetic inheritance, and its reliance on the digital imagination of intelligence as information, occludes the actual modes in which biology and its organic basis matters in human reproduction, particularly as these modes and functions are still being actively discovered.

Feminist anthropologists and science studies scholars lead us to ask how the organizing metaphors through which we conceive of the body and its processes tie into the formation of social and power relationships. Technologies and their refiguring of bodies are never neutral, and in fact that metaphorizing of the body embeds it with histories of power (Star 1991) and invests it with empowered worldviews (Haraway 1997, 11). The mechanical body and the socially embedded notion of the passive femininity of pregnancy come together as part of a worldview in which an artificial uterus for the gestation of the human embryo and fetus makes sense, and by extension enables the logic of renting the uterus of a female human being for the same purpose.

Like the mechanized body and the functional view of organs as separable parts of that body, the shift in obstetrics from a focus on maternal outcome to fetal outcome is also a necessary component of the history of possibility for commercial surrogacy (Martin 2001, 64). For example, Emily Martin has traced the evolution of the metaphor of the body as an industrial society as it evolved alongside the historical process of industrialization. The metaphor extends from the level of the cell as a factory up through the flexibilization of global production and the concomitant model of the flexible body elaborated through metaphors describing the immune system (Martin 1995). She sums up the metaphors in obstetrics texts as "juxtaposing two pictures: the uterus as a machine that produces the baby and the woman as laborer who produces the baby" (2001, 65). The doctor is seen as "the supervisor or foreman of the labor process" (Ibid.). As a potentially productive, but unused part, the uterus of the potential surrogate offends capitalist sensibilities (Ibid., 45). As someone who lacks a genetic relationship to the fetus, the Indian surrogate is positioned within the structure of international fertility travel as providing a service to the commissioning parents as the owner of a uterus that is a space and machine to be let out and whose production is to be professionally managed (Vora 2013), producing a new type of mother-worker subject (Pande 2014).

Commercial surrogacy, like other practices in ART and biotechnology, relies on the use of technologies to reorganize, or reconceptualize the body as a site of potential productivity. A common narration of the bodily phenomenon of commercial surrogacy that gets related in both ethnographic accounts and media accounts is that it is renting the use of an organ for a limited time (Vora 2009, 2012; Winddance-Twine 2011; Pande 2014). Imagined as an empty space, or as an unused object separate from the organic functioning of the body, the womb-for-rent and the woman who is surrogate become interchangeable in both public discourse and in much of legal and medical policy, as she gets erased as a medical subject other than as a gestational carrier, and is limited in action by contractual restrictions on decisions about her body while pregnant (Vora 2012; Saravanan 2013; Pande 2014). Social scientists studying surrogacy have explained that surrogacy in India has been stigmatized as bodily labor (Pande 2010; Saravanan 2013), and as delimited as a 9-month work contract (Pande 2014). Understanding how surrogacy is connected to the scientific imagination of the uterus as an isolated and necessary "part" for the biological reproduction of humans offers additional context for the low compensation for surrogacy, the relatively low social value for this work, and the lack of attention in Indian national policy to the need for long-term entitlements for women who have been surrogates. Identifying the biological fallacy of this understanding of gestation may offer tools to destabilize the effects of this imagination in the determination of legal protections for former surrogates.

The imagination of the uterus as separate from the biology and subject of the human body is a historical product. During the 1990s and early 2000s, scientists in the United States and Japan were conducting a range of experiments involving the creation of artificial uterine environments. Japanese scientists developed an acrylic womb in late 1992, and in the United States there were experiments with growing uterine tissue on the curved internal surface of nonorganic containers as possible ex vivo gestational environments (Klass 1996; McKie 2002; Reynolds 2005). These efforts were modestly successful in getting nonhuman mammal embryos to attach and grow for several weeks. However, eventually the project of creating an artificial womb was given up, and subsequent research has shown that the influence of the maternal environment on fetal development is so complex that the creation of an artificial uterus is no longer seen as a worthwhile endeavor. How and why did scientific communities come to a place in history where a uterus outside of the body could be imagined, even desired, and how did it come to be perceived as a significant need in an arguably unsustainably growing human population?

The social impact of fetal imaging has been rigorously tracked by scholars (Kevles 1998; Rapp 1999; Stabile 1998), beginning with the famous April 30, 1965, Life cover story entitled "Drama of Life Before Birth," which contained photographs described as "the first portraits ever made of a living embryo inside its mother's womb." Tracing the impact of fetal imaging on the presence of the maternal body in media representations and popular imagination, Carole Stabile notes that in these 1965 images the mother is "shot through" but doesn't need to be completely erased (1998, 178). She explains that following *Roe v. Wade* (1973), the stakes of controlling the pregnant woman's body are raised with the legal establishment of a woman's reproductive choice, resulting in the need to eliminate the maternal body from visualizing technologies and public discourse in favor of exclusive focus on the fetus as patient, subject, or citizen. Just as fetal personhood relies on the erasure of the maternal body and the reduction of pregnant women to passive reproductive machines (172), the autonomy of commissioning parents in surrogacy agreements relies on the erasure of the gestational surrogate's active role as a potential parental subject or genetic author of the future child. This passive role for the surrogate is advocated in current surrogacy contracts and draft ART legislation in India.

Geneticization, the process by which genetics has come to explain health and disease, and to naturalize social differences as biologically based (Lippman 1991), also operates in ART practice to naturalize genetic descent as legitimate parentage, and egg donors and surrogates as providers of what Cooper and Waldby call " 'services in the self': services that rely on in vivo, biological processing and the utilization of the worker's living substrate as essential elements in the productive process" (2014, 65). This results in the expectation that surrogates become entrepreneurial subjects, taking on the work of self-management that allows them to perform contracted surrogacy. This includes, "consent to the constitution of her uterus as an asset class, able to generate monopoly rent," effectively renting her "excess reproductive capacity," as these "must remain in vivo," and so the commissioning parents must establish their rights to this remote biology through lease" (Ibid., 84).

Women who participate in surrogacy have not described their role as simply or as one-dimensionally as have social representations of the womb-for-rent and their medical and legal corollaries. For example, Pande's ethnography underlines surrogates' narratives of the influence of their blood on the developing infant (2009), and my own ethnography relates narratives that emphasize the necessarily enduring connection between surrogates and commissioning families that defy the genetic logic of connection as existing only between commissioning parents and infant (Vora 2015). The medical and legal practices involved in commercial gestational surrogacy, as well as the ethics of how participants make decisions about their participation, are guided by often divergent understandings of such figures as the gene, the fetus, and the uterus as isolated from, or metonymic with, the surrogate as a pregnant female body. Refiguration, or contesting the meaning of figures like the gene or fetus, therefore becomes a site of political potential.

One example of a site for the potential refiguration of the role of the uterus in gestation from being an alienable part of the passive, machinic pregnant body could be in the active research on fetal-cell microchimerism in immunology. A growing body of immunological research explores the exchange of cells between a pregnant woman and fetus during pregnancy. This exchange occurs in both directions between the fetus and the mother, and fetal cells continue to circulate in the mother's body for years after pregnancy (Hird 2007, 9). Chimerism refers to the presence of two genetically distinct cell lines (genomes) in an organism, and fetal-cell microchimerism describes the cellular interchange between the pregnant woman and the fetus. As Susan Elizabeth Kelly notes, the discovery of this phenomenon challenges the notion of the immune self, the basic tenet of immunology (2012, 246). But on an ontological level, it also "challenges previous biological understandings of a barrier between the body of a pregnant woman and the developing foetus, a barrier maintaining the identity integrity as it were, of two beings, two separate subjects," thus contesting the understanding of individuals as discretely bound organisms (Ibid., 234). Aryn Martin argues that the practices of scientists (biologists and clinicians) who research feto-maternal microchimerism "don't simply study, describe, or reveal the phenomenon, but rather they usher the phenomenon into being—in particular ways and not others—through their imaginations, practices, and language" (2010, 32). Martin looks to the scientific challenge of microchimerism to offer a promise for feminist materialisms and biologies, as it suggests that "within our tissues and organs entities exist simultaneously that have been characterized as mutually exclusive: self/other, male/female, child/adult, black/white, and so on." (2010, 41).

Since a maternal body may contain cells exchanged through previous pregnancies as well as with her own gestational mother (Hird 2007, 9), she becomes a node in a multigenerational and multibodied exchange of genetically different cells (Guettier et al. 2005). For gestational surrogacy, whose basic model of legal parental rights is mediated through geneticism and property (Vora 2012), the disturbance of the nature-culture category of biosocial selves could provide scientific grounds for arguments made by surrogates about their influence, through pregnancy, on the developing fetus, and the timeline of the effect of the maternal and fetal bodies upon one another, perhaps offering the potential for an ontological shift that would enable more equitable long-term provisions for current and former surrogates.

In embryology labs and fertility clinics, practitioners work toward manifesting worldviews into futures, worldviews that imagine away the body and nurture-work of the so-called gestational carrier in favor of the empty uterus, the isolated fetus, the heroic doctor, and the intended parents. In these moments, such worldviews suggest how participants can be networked into these imagined futures, and how they cannot. In other words, in addition to seeing new physical relationships forming between bodies, and between technological instruments and bodies in the ART clinic, we also see a contest over how new socialities are forming around the technologies (Pande 2009, 2014; Vora 2014, 2015; Deomampo 2014). However, just as emerging research on the complex role of the maternal environment undermined the scientific worldview and experiments in building an artificial womb, research pointing to the genetic importance of the gestational mother's body has the potential to destabilize the division between the gestational body and the surrogate as a genetic individual with influence on the fetal body, a role that threatens the segregated authorship of the commissioning parents. At the least, such destabilizing of the genetic individual would have the potential to shift how we imagine the role of the maternal body as passive, which aligns with the arguments by women in India who have been through surrogacy that the role of the surrogate is active and authorial in producing the eventual infant she bears.

Creative Authorship, Service Work, and the Gendered Body

Despite techno-utopic projections like that represented by the artificial uterus, the body and labor-power continue to be irreplaceable commodities. The instruments of production of postindustrial life include the very bodies of producers in expanded ways, and subjects may be coerced into using them up in the act of production. Service or care, and its circulation as a form of labor, connects the current growth of the commercial surrogacy industry in India to a longer history of the biopolitics of outsourcing, and before that colonialism, in their connecting of Indians to transnational economics. Gendered divisions of labor in both the sphere of industry and the sphere of the heteropatriarchal family come together in the clinic mapped on to bodies that have been prefigured by colonial and other histories of difference. The commissioning parents are situated to take advantage of transnational surrogacy arrangements as the result of their own stratified histories, and as such bring those histories to bear upon their connection to India and the contracted relationship to the surrogate.

The historical gendering of the pregnant female body as a passive vessel is part of a larger structure of understanding that feminizes actions and roles deemed noncreative or noninnovative. Even before the technological interventions discussed above, the body of the pregnant woman was culturally constructed as a passive object:

> in the mother-to-be the antithesis of subject and object ceases to exist; she and the child with which she is swollen make up together an equivalent pair overwhelmed by life. Ensnared by nature, the pregnant woman is plant and animal . . . she is a human being, a conscious and free individual, who has become life's passive instrument.
>
> (de Beauvoir 1949 [1972], 512–513)

The feminized subjects performing domestic work and childcare in the heteropatriarchal private sphere were gendered as such as the result of a historical process that created a new subject, the housewife. The housewife did domestic and care work out of love, according to Maria Mies, with the love also being a historical construct (1986).

Feminist theories have shown that the subject of labor power, the presumed male worker in the public sphere, relies on a host of supports that originate in the vital energy of others, supports that do not appear to be labor or behave like it. These include the historical structure of the Protestant heteropatriarchal household with its wife, children, and servants (Mies 1986; Jakobsen 2013). The role of the pregnant woman's body in commercial gestational surrogacy as passive object relies on a fundamental understanding of creative authorship as gendered, and upon the distinction between authorial, masculine discovery/invention and feminine, reproductive, servile support labor. In cases where the intended parent and gamete donor are not the same, the discourse of "intention" trumps the discourse of genetics in identifying the rightful parents of the infant-to-be. In Indian gestational surrogacy as represented by the Draft ART Bill and Rules (2012), the genetic noninvolvement of the surrogate justifies her social and legal exclusion from the world of intended parents.

In biological and biotechnological research and development, and in genetic therapy research and development in particular, there are very particular notions of what counts as invention, and these are engaged with legal protections of intellectual patent and property. Laws protecting intellectual property rely upon historically gendered notions of active versus passive creativity, where "support" labor, like that performed by nonauthorial lower class hired workers or embodied or physical production, does not figure as producing property, and is therefore not recognized as an invention or the result of creative labor. The woman who enters a surrogacy contract under current conditions in India, given the histories discussed above, enters as a service provider whose support labor is designated as passive and noncreative in both frameworks of labor and of private property.

Effects of Embodied Inequality in Fertility Travel and Surrogacy Practice

Rather than a passive vessel or object of masculine authorial reproduction marked by DNA, the maternal body in immunological research on fetal-cell microchimerism suggests a different potential set of metaphors for re-evaluating the role of the pregnant body, and therefore the role of the surrogate, in fertility service economies like that in India. However, present remuneration for surrogacy is based on the common sense devaluation of the mechanical and passive pregnant body, and the uterus as rentable part. As labor, surrogacy is devalued as service and reproductive work through the international division of labor and its colonial roots as they play out in trade agreements like GATS and legislation like the Draft ART Bill and Rules (2012) in India that protect relatively powerful consumers over producers of services (Cooper and Waldby 2014). However, for the present, given the reliance of fertility travel to India upon the potentiality of bodies as produced through histories of inequality and instrumentalization, there are a number of conclusions to draw.

Discursively, the womb as a detached commodity circulated in a transnational market removes the surrogate as a subject of medicine. It also places surrogacy and the women performing it under the domain of market-based legal values, which protect consumers and property owners. In a market scenario like this, the surrogate becomes a womb, or a carrier, interchangeable as an anonymous commodity (Knoch 2014), rather than as a subject of human rights, of law, or of medicine. This "co-optation of the maternal into a sole economic understanding of women's bodies" plays into existing national and international hierarchies of race, class and gender" (Riggs and Due 2010, 22).

The current draft law regulating ART practice in India governs actors through market-based rights that favor commissioning parents as consumers. A surrogate does not have any say regarding practices like embryo reduction and cesarian deliveries beyond her agreement with the clinic's general policy (SAMA 2012), and there is currently no state recognition of any legally defensible connection between the surrogate and her direct family with the child to whom she gives birth. The infant is not a contracting party and therefore his/her interests are not represented (Ibid., 27). Until the expected future codification of their rights in Indian legislation, the contracting or intended parents are vulnerable subjects as they negotiate the legal meaning of parentage between national legal structures and ARTs. There are clear legal and medical interventions to be made to decrease inequality and risk for vulnerable actors in fertility travel, but given India's involvement with the WTO and GATS, the interests of the market are likely to remain a primary influence. In light of this, SAMA: Organization for Women's Health's report on surrogacy concludes that what is needed by surrogates is legal aid and counseling throughout the recruitment and surrogacy process, as well as advocacy for rights of surrogates (SAMA 2012, 43). In addition to the potentially adverse health outcomes for surrogates and infants born through surrogacy, there are long-term social consequences for all participants that are only beginning to be understood (Knoch 2014), even as short-term consequences like custody and immigration problems are still being worked out through national courts in India and in the home countries of commissioning parents.

Conclusion

India's colonial history and its influence on the evolution of India's role in the globalized international division of labor are part of the background for the development of medical tourism to India. Practicing a postcolonial focus in thinking through the role of new technologies, such as those in ART creating the conditions for medical travel to India for IVF and surrogacy, means bracketing the newness of the technologies in favor of a focus on their historical continuities. India's national emphasis on science and technology education following independence and the practice of nonresident Indians seeking medical care on return trips to India combine with a larger pattern in decolonizing nations of skipping over Fordist production and industrialization and joining the global economy in the mode of post-Fordism. Subaltern and postcolonial studies approaches to medicine in colonial India have also explained the way that in such an economic climate, the suppression of indigenous interests is common in the development of social and economic policies that advance the interests of economically and politically dominant classes (Arnold 1993; Prakash 1999). As Marcia Inhorn has shown, the vast difference in material conditions between women in the population of surrogacy providers and those of the surrogacy consumers (both in India and internationally) mean that what is newly developed or arrived in India may be largely unnecessary for the local population, and in fact may become mainly a tool for the expropriation of value or services for a foreign or elite Indian consuming population (2003). The social structure of this situation means that there is not a one-dimensional feminist approach for the study of the role of scientific knowledge and new technologies in fertility travel, and the analysis of fertility travel to India must be set in the longer history of how science, medicine, and technology have been involved in India's history.

Bringing together the role that medicine and medical education have played in India's colonial and postcolonial history with the origins of the notion of the instrumentalized uterus, part of a cultural imagination of mind-body separation, and more specifically, the body as a machine composed of parts, helps to explain the way that surrogacy and those who perform it in

India become devalued economically and legally. The notions of the private individual body as a medical and social object derive from an ongoing historical relationship whereby other modes of embodiment and sociality are influenced and overwritten through institutions like the ART clinic and technologies that enact fantasies based on the biological, genetic individual, and the individuality of the labor contract engaged in surrogacy. The preoccupation with the body as property in the protections offered to surrogates in the Draft ART Bill and Rules (2012) are also part of this process, which DasGupta and Dasgupta argue is not congruent with the relational and collective emphasis in Indian culture (2015, 140).[2] However, as Amrita Pande points out, discourses of ownership of the body can be empowering as well, giving women a place from which to assert decisions about reproduction and sexuality, as well as a way to substantiate their contribution to household income (2014, 251).

Research like that on fetal-cell microchimerism that expands our understanding of the biological relationship between maternal and fetal bodies, and challenges the notion of the genetic individual, has the potential to denaturalize the isolation of the uterus as simply a functional machinic part of a woman's passive biological reproductivity. This understanding of the gendered body has repercussions for Indian surrogates, whose financial compensation, health care, and legal isolation from the commissioning parent and infant is influenced by the equating of women who perform surrogacy with their instrumentalized function as temporary gestational carriers. At the least, such destabilizing of the genetic individual would have the potential to shift how we imagine the role of the maternal body as passive, which aligns with the arguments by women in India who have been through surrogacy that the role of the surrogate is active and authorial in producing the eventual infant she bears.

Notes

1 The vast gap in resources between producers and consumers in the transnational surrogacy clinic engages histories of power and difference established in India's colonial history, and therefore requires attention to the relations of power established by the surrogacy contract, but also to the particular forms of dependency in established by the surrogacy contract. the current absence of regulation in India means contractual arrangements may contain incomplete or absent information. Consent, and therefore autonomy, is thus incomplete despite being arranged through a freely entered agreement (Vora 2012).

2 Cited by Pande 2014, 250.

Works Cited

Arnold, David. (1988). "Touching the Body: Perspectives on the Indian Plague," in *Selected Subaltern Studies*, R. Guha and G. Chakravorty Spivak, eds. New Delhi: Oxford University Press, pp. 391–426.

Arnold, David. (1993). *Colonizing the Body*. Berkeley and Los Angeles: University of California Press.

Braidotti, Rosi. (2013). *The Posthuman*. Cambridge: Polity.

Cartwright, Lisa. (1995). *Screening the Body: Tracing Medicine's Visual Culture*. Minneapolis, MA: University of Minnesota Press.

Cooper, Melinda and Catherine Waldby. (2014). *Clinical Labor: Tissue Donors and Research Subjects in the Global Bioeconomy*. Durham, NC: Duke University Press.

DasGupta, Sayantani and Shamita Das Dasgupta. (2015). "Business as Usual? The Violence of Reproductive Trafficking in the Indian Context," in *Globalization and Transnational Surrogacy in India: Outsourcing Life*, DasGupta, Sayantani and Shamita Das Dasgupta, eds. pp. 179–196.

de Beauvoir, Simone. *The Second Sex*. (1949 [1972]). translated by H. M. Parshley. New York: Penguin. 512–513.

Deomampo, Daisy. (2013). "Gendered Geographies of Reproductive Tourism," *Gender & Society*, 27(4): 514–527.

Deomampo, Daisy. (2014). "Defining Parents, Making Citizens: Nationality and Citizenship in Transnational Surrogacy," *Medical Anthropology: Cross-Cultural Studies in Health and Illness*, 1–16.

Derbyshire, David. (2004). "Woman Gives Birth to Her Grandchildren," *The Telegraph*, January 30. www.telegraph.co.uk/news/worldnews/asia/india/1453012/Woman-gives-birth-to-her-grandchildren.html. Accessed April 1, 2009.

Francis, Sabil. (2001). "The IITs in India: Symbols of an Emerging Nation," *South Asia Chronicle*, 1: 293–326.

Guettier, C., M. Sebagh, J. Buard, D. Feneux, M. Ortin-Serrano, M. Gigou, V. Tricottet, M. Reyne, D. Samuel and C. Fe'ray. (2005). "Male Cell Microchimerism in Normal and Diseased Female Livers from Foetal Life to Adulthood," *Hepatology*, 42(1): 35–43 (cited by Kelly 2012, 243).

Haraway, Donna. (1997). *ModestWitness@Second_Millennium.Female-Man_Meets_OncoMouse: Feminism and Technoscience*. New York: Routledge.

Hird, Myra J. (2007). "The Corporeal Generosity of Maternity," *Body & Society*, 13(1): 1–20.

Hochschild, Arlie. (2012). *The Outsourced Self*. New York: Metropolitan Books, Henry Holt and Company LLC.

Inhorn, M.C. (2003). "Global Infertility and the Globalization of New Reproductive Technologies: Illustrations from Egypt," *Social Science & Medicine*, 56: 1837–1851.

Inhorn, Marcia C. (2012). "Reproductive Exile in Global Dubai: South Asian Stories," *Cultural Politics*, 8: 283–306.

Jakobsen, Janet. (2013). "Perverse Justice," *GLQ: A Journal of Lesbian and Gay Studies*, 18(1): 25.

Kambli, Raelene. (2011). "IVF in India: The Story so Far . . .," *Financial Express*, December. http://healthcare.financialexpress.com/201112/market01.shtml. Accessed April 12, 2014.

Kelly, Susan Elizabeth. (2012). "The Maternal-Foetal Interface and Gestational Chimerism: The Emerging Importance of Chimeric Bodies," *Science as Culture*, 21(2): 233–257.

Kevles, B. (1998). *Naked to the Bone: Medical Imaging in the Twentieth Century*. Reading, MA: Addison-Wesley.

Klass, Perri. (1996). "The Artificial Womb Is Born," *The New York Times*, September 29. www.nytimes.com/1996/09/29/magazine/the-artificial-womb-is-born.html. Accessed March 1, 2013.

Knoch, Jonathan K. (2014). "Health Concerns and Ethnical Considerations Regarding International Surrogacy," *International Journal of Gynecology & Obstetrics*, April 27. www.sciencedirect.com/science/article/pii/S0020729214002276. Accessed May 15, 2014.

Lippman, Abby. (1991). "Prenatal Genetic Testing and Screening: Constructing Needs and Reinforcing Inequalities," *American Journal of Law and Medicine*, 17(1–2): 15–50.

Martin, Aryn. (2010). "'Your Mother's Always with You': Material Feminism and Fetomaternal Microchimerism," *Resources for Feminist Research*, 33(3–4): 31.

Martin, Emily. (1995). *Flexible Bodies*. Boston, MA: Beacon Press.

Martin, Emily. (2001). *The Woman in the Body: A Cultural Analysis of Reproduction*. Boston, MA: Beacon Press.

McKie, Robin. (2002). "Men Redundant? Now We Don't Need Women Either," *The Guardian*, February 10. www.theguardian.com/world/2002/feb/10/medicalscience.research. Accessed March 1, 2013.

Mies, Maria. (1986). *Patriarchy and Accumulation on a World Scale: Women in the International Division of Labor*. London: Third World Books; Atlantic Highlands, NJ: Zed Books, Distributed in the U.S.A. and Canada by Humanities Press.

Pande, Amrita. (2009). "It May Be Her Eggs but It Is My Blood: Surrogates and Everyday Forms of Kinship in India," *Qualitative Sociology*, 32(4): 379–397.

Pande, Amrita. (2010). "Commercial Surrogacy in India: Manufacturing a Perfect Mother-Worker," *Signs: Journal of Women in Culture and Society*, 35(4): 969–994.

Pande, Amrita. (2014). *Wombs in Labor: Transnational Commercial Surrogacy in India*. New York: Columbia University Press.

Parks, J. (2010). "Care Ethics and the Global Practice of Commercial Surrogacy," *Bioethics*, 24(7): 333–340.

Prakash, Gyan. (1999). *Another Reason: Science and the Imagination of Modern India*. Princeton, NJ: Princeton University Press.

Prashad, Vijay. (2007). *The Darker Nations: A People's History of the Third World*. New York: The New Press.

Rapp, R. (1999). *Testing Women, Testing the Fetus: The Social Impact of Amniocentesis in America*. New York: Routledge.

Reynolds, Gretchen. (2005). "Artificial Wombs: Will We Grow Babies Outside of the Mothers Bodies?," *Popular Science*, August 1. www.popsci.com/scitech/article/2005-08/artificial-wombs. Accessed March 1, 2013.

Riggs, D.W. and C. Due. (2010). "Gay Men, Race Privilege and Surrogacy in India," *Outskirts: Feminisms Along the Edge*, 22.

Rudrappa, S. (2012). "Working India's Reproduction Assembly Line: Surrogacy and Reproductive Rights?" *Western Humanities Review*, 66(3): 77.

SAMA: Resource Group for Women's Health. (2012). *Birthing a Market: A Study on Commercial Surrogacy*. New Delhi: SAMA. www.samawomenshealth.org/downloads/Birthing%20A%20Market.pdf.

Saravanan, Sheela. (2013). "An Ethnomethodological Approach to Examine Exploitation in the Context of Capacity, Trust and Experience of Commercial Surrogacy in India," *Philosophy, Ethics, and Humanities in Medicine*, 8: 10.

Stabile, C. (1998). "Shooting the Mother: Fetal Photography and the Politics of Disappearance," in *The Visible Woman: Imaging Technologies, Gender, and Science*, P.A. Treichler, L. Cartwright and C. Penley, eds. New York: New York University Press.

Star, Susan Leigh. (1991). "Power, Technology, and the Phenomenology of Conventions: On Being Allergic to Onions," in *A Sociology of Monsters: Essays on Power, Technology, and Domination*, J. Law, ed. London and New York: Routledge, pp. 26–56.

Towghi, Fouzieyha and Kalindi Vora. (2014). "Bodies, Markets and the Experimental in South Asia," *Ethnos: Journal of Anthropology*, 79(1): 1–18.

Vora, Kalindi. (2009). "Indian Transnational Surrogacy and the Commodification of Vital Energy," *Subjectivities*, 28(1): 266–278.

Vora, Kalindi. (2012). "Limits of Labor," *South Atlantic Quarterly*, 201(111): 681–700.

Vora, Kalindi. (2013). "Potential, Risk and Return in Transnational Indian Gestational Surrogacy," *Current Anthropology*, 54(suppl. 7): S97–S105.

Vora, Kalindi. (2014). "Experimental Socialities and Gestational Surrogacy in the Indian ART Clinic," *Ethnos: Journal of Anthropology*, 79(1): 63–83.

Vora, Kalindi. (2015). *Life Support: Biocapital and the New History of Outsourced Labor*. Minneapolis, MA: University of Minnesota Press.

Wallerstein, Immanuel Maurice. (1976). *The Modern World-System: Capitalist Agriculture and the Origins of the European World-Economy in the Sixteenth Century*. New York: Academic Press.

Winddance-Twine, Francis. (2011). *Outsourcing the Womb: Race, Class and Gestational Surrogacy in a Global Market*. London: Routledge.

6

POTENTIAL, RISK, AND RETURN IN TRANSNATIONAL INDIAN GESTATIONAL SURROGACY

Growing transnational demand for technological intervention in conception and gestation, combined with the unregulated status of assisted reproductive technology (ART) clinics in India, has resulted in rapidly growing numbers of ART clinics serving transnational and wealthy Indian clientele. This essay focuses on how participants, including surrogates, commissioning parents, physicians, and clinic staff, attach meaning to bodies and relationships mediated through ARTs. I argue that the bodies of women are potentialized to become both surrogates and a locus for new social meaning by the availability of ARTs and highly trained physicians in a location where there is minimal regulatory oversight and where women's material context makes surrogacy a financial necessity. The relationship between physical bodies and social meaning becomes oriented toward seemingly multiple future outcomes when surrogates use the continuous shift between economic and interpersonal registers in the clinic to imagine a long-term beneficial connection to commissioning parents. The politics that position the clinic to potentialize the bodies of surrogates, and the way participants imagine the outcomes of relationships established in the clinic, occur at a moment in which India has both highly educated medical professionals with access to cutting-edge technology as well as a large population of people without access to sufficient resources. As such, the potentializing of women's bodies as gestational surrogates relies on differentiation of subjects culturally, geographically, and economically. While the goal of gestational surrogacy may be straightforward in the eyes of the commissioning parties (the production of an infant), the way that various participants understand the process and its resulting social relations—both current and future—are multiple. This article examines several ways in which the potentializing of bodies and resulting social relations are negotiated as participants navigate the uncharted terrain of transnational gestational surrogacy.

The largely unrestricted ART clinic in India was produced through an accident of historical conjunctures and has been encouraged in growth by a transnational and primarily urban-based Indian consuming class's willingness to seize a moment of possibility. The clinic is a productive place

DOI: 10.4324/9781003353362-6

in which to observe, as Taussig et al. (2013) state, several "processes of becoming." Tracking these processes is valuable because they offer a site in which to observe the "articulations and practices" through which diverse participants negotiate "the task of being simultaneously biological things and human persons" in the face of "moral claims that emerging medical technologies make on people's bodies" (Taussig et al. 2013). The social structures and material conditions at work within the clinic shape the ways that actors negotiate their relationships with one another; processes that through the lens of potentiality can be seen to work to secure an otherwise uncertain situation.

This essay uses observation and interviews from fieldwork in the Manushi clinic, consideration of the proposed ART Bill and Rules currently under discussion in the Indian parliament, and the work of anthropologists, activists, and theorists to examine the ways that risk and expectation of future return motivates participants. These participants must navigate between risk and expectation in relation to how they understand the social relations formed through the clinic (see also Simpson, this volume). In the first section, I address the ART policies and practices of the clinic, including its general geographic and political context, showing how many social and economic relations are up for negotiation even as the clinic's basic medical practices are well-established. I then turn to the ways the bodies of women as surrogates are potentialized through narrative and other forms of representation at the clinic, including scientific discourse, in combination with sharp differences in access to resources. The third section turns directly to the expectations of both surrogates and commissioning parents. Here, the stories both parties tell point to a wide gap in the imagined potential created through the clinic as well as risks these participants take in pursuit of the promise of future reward or rewards. The rewards may be both financial and altruistic for surrogates, including a hope by some for long-term connection with commissioning parents. For commissioning parents, the reward is an infant that shares meaningful biological qualities, including genetics; and for the directors of this particular clinic, the rewards are financial gain coupled with the representation of responsible conduct toward concerned parties. In the final section, I build on the discussion of risk and examine the clinic's description of the ways it "rehabilitates" the surrogates as an example of how participants negotiate registers of altruistic and economic relations as they work to secure their preferred outcomes for the potentiality raised in the context of the clinic.

The Potentializing Clinic

ART clinics in India are currently expected to follow national guidelines, but are not subject to regulatory laws. This means that individual clinics can form idiosyncratic policies regarding practice based on discretionary adherence to these guidelines, with only the market and the management's sense of responsibility and ethics limiting what a clinic can offer and what arrangements it might make. There exists current draft legislation, but it does not define reporting or surveillance instruments for the regulations it proposes, and so it is unclear how long it will be before clinics must follow uniformly applied and enforced rules. In the context of the rapid social change taking place in India, and the transnational commissioning parents entering surrogacy contracts with Indian women, this potentializing of women's bodies as surrogates also creates a unique social context in which participants can imagine multiple outcomes for their relationships. I argue that the social relations and economic opportunities that emerge from the social and financial practice in the under-regulated clinic are heavily influenced by commitments that clinics make to promoting and enforcing the meanings attached to relationships formed through surrogacy arrangements in the clinic, as well as the limits on economic activity proposed in national legislation intended to regulate the industry.

After the Manushi clinic's first successful surrogacy case in the early 2000s and the resultant media attention, demand led the clinic—which then and still operates primarily as a standard OB/GYN practice catering to local patients—to begin hiring increasing numbers of self-referred surrogates. A set of clinic policies formed organically over time, and by 2008, when I observed the clinic and conducted interviews, the experience for most surrogates, and to a lesser extent commissioning parents, had been standardized. For example, when a client herself does not have viable eggs, eggs from Indian donors are used; the clinic stipulates that the surrogate and the donor must be separate individuals, both of whom the clinic selects without input from commissioning couples. After an initial interview, there is usually little contact between surrogate mothers and commissioning parents. The clinic houses surrogates in hostels that their family members may visit if they live close enough to do so; few of the surrogates originally come from the town where the clinic is located. Surrogates are said to receive a fee of roughly US $6000, which can be the equivalent of up to 9 years of their regular family income. The overall surrogacy process at this clinic costs clients about US $20 000, in comparison to the US $80 000–100 000 it can cost in the United States.

At the Manushi clinic there is a policy of permitting only single or twin pregnancies for the protection of the mother and remaining fetus(es). The clinic also mandates that surrogates be married with at least one child, both to prove the viability of her uterus and because the directors believe it makes attachment to the commissioned infant less likely.[1] While these self-imposed policies are uncontroversial, there have been stories in the news in India of unwed women undertaking surrogacy, a concept culturally scandalous enough to provoke a public reaction, as well as pregnancy with multiples greater than twins, and of other culturally or legally dubious practices.

Doctors at the Manushi clinic and commissioning parents who had chosen this clinic after visiting others in nearby cities mentioned that some of these other clinics seemed nontransparent and "fishy," and anecdotal evidence suggests that many more clinics are performing surrogacy arrangements than are advertising them.

Just as the Manushi clinic's ART policies and practices were formed as needed and with little standardization, social relationships appear similarly unstructured. The brief account below provides a sense of the comparatively informal and sometimes ad hoc nature of organization and social relations in the clinic. It sketches a scene in which social relations between doctors, commissioning parents, staff, and surrogates are in flux and open to negotiation as a result of the potentializing of women's bodies as surrogates.

I sat in one of the clinic's two office rooms one day as Dr. H., co-director of the clinic, described the typical process for the increasing number of foreigners going through the stages of egg harvesting and semen collection towards gestational surrogacy via in vitro fertilization (IVF).[2] Listening in to our conversation was David, a commissioning father from the United States who was visiting without his wife and was in the early stages of IVF and gestational surrogacy using donor eggs. Also present was Sanjay, a commissioning father and a nonresident Indian from the United Kingdom with extended family in the region, whose twins had been born by a surrogate a few days earlier. Sanjay had met one of the clinic directors at a public lecture about the clinic in the United Kingdom several years prior, and had been in touch with the directors since that time. Dr. H. said that after the administration of hormones and later inducement to ovulation for the commissioning mother (or for the egg donor in the case that the commissioning mother's eggs are not being used), an egg is fertilized and an embryo is cultured with the goal of transferring it to the uterus of the surrogate. He noted that on day 2 of the culture, parents can view an embryo under the microscope, and that when an embryo is transferred, the (commissioning) mother may attend the procedure, though he did not mention how the preference of the surrogate mother figured into this decision.[3] As we were talking, additional visitors came and left the office and engaged in short conversations with Dr H. or others in the room.

Following up on a comment he had made the previous day that surrogate mothers at Manushi, and in India generally, are "different than in the West," Dr. H. elaborated that the purpose for becoming a surrogate mother is different for women in India. He said, "women enter into surrogacy because of the desire to earn money to start a small business or educate their children. In that sense, their decision concerns the well-being of their whole family." His impression was that women who become surrogates elsewhere desire to earn spending money for consumables or leisure-time activities. He had previously explained that the clinic makes a practice of holding the fees earned by a surrogate until she is ready to use them toward a specific end.

The reason he gave was that if the men in her family get a hold of the fee, "they will spend it on a new motorbike or on drinking, and even the women who aren't necessarily that educated, will spend it on elaborate religious celebrations." He explained that the clinic has made all of the financial interactions in the clinic transparent.

Ajay, the driver for the clinic and sometimes tour guide for guests walked in to ask Dr. H. about the schedule for an arriving client. After he left, Dr. H. explained to David that Ajay spoke functional English. David mentioned that he would be interested in paying Ajay extra money to take him sightseeing. David then asked Dr. H. if he could change money there on premises, which Dr. H. did within a few minutes. Sanjay joked that the clinic is also a currency exchange. After some time, a man came in to get a stack of paperwork from Dr. H., who followed him out of the room. Sanjay offered that this man manages all of the birth certificates for infants born by surrogates to foreign commissioning parents, noting that, "he can get things done in two hours that would take me three weeks." Sanjay implied that the man (whom I later found out is also a nonmedical assistant in the surgery theater) has some sort of internal connections in several Mumbai embassies. Later in the afternoon, a woman who had just agreed to become a surrogate came in to sign some paperwork. After she departed, Dr. H. said, "You do a surrogate mother's [intake] interview and you get a vibe—good or not. I get a good vibe from her, that she will carry the baby successfully." Dr. B., the co-director of the clinic, came in a little later and announced in English that David, who was also in the room, had three good embryos for transfer. She added in Gujarati, to Dr. H., that because of his advanced age (in his early to mid-fifties) she had to create a high number of embryos. Dr. H. nodded in my direction, a gesture that I assumed was to remind her that I could follow the conversation, unlike David. Another surrogate mother who was not introduced to me came in a few minutes later to receive her second trimester payment. Entering the conversation after sitting quietly for more than 45 minutes, and perhaps in response to the informality he perceived in the clinic, David said that he was afraid someone "[would] shut the clinic down" before his surrogate delivers.

The above interactions, all taking place in one room of the clinic on the same day, illustrate not only the informal economies and inchoate relations in play, but also the way that attachment of meaning to the social relations formed through the clinic work toward desired outcomes. I argue that this interplay is the direct result of attempts by different participants to secure future outcomes based on competing notions of what those should be.

Bodies and Sociality

To begin to approach the social, economic, and ethical factors influencing the outcome of the potentialized bodies and the creation of social relations around them represented in the transnational ART clinic in India, I will examine some of the bodily concepts in play in the context of this clinic. These include conceptions of the body as described by surrogates, commissioning parents, and doctors and other staff in the clinic. Women who become surrogates are first made potential surrogates by a combination of their financial needs and lack of other resources, as well as the technologies that make surrogacy through IVF possible for commissioning parents. In addition, I will attend to how the discourses managing how the meaning of the bodily process of gestation, as well as gametes from commissioning parents and/or paid donors, matter to the relationships between participants in the clinic and influence different understandings of what outcomes should result from participation as commissioning parent or surrogate.

The surrogates I spoke to, including former and current surrogates and women waiting hopefully to find out if they had become pregnant as surrogates, first described surrogacy to me in the manner they assumed I wanted to hear, as it was what clinic staff, doctors, and former surrogates counseled them to understand and accept: the uterus is a space in a woman's body that is empty when she is not expecting a child, and surrogacy is simply the renting out of that space for someone else's child (see also Vora 2009; Pande 2009). The empty uterus is also that which is emphasized in headlines across the world sensationalizing transnational commercial surrogacy as "wombs for rent."[4] Surrogates at Manushi clinic described the effort to become a gestational carrier in terms of managing who knows about their pregnancy, of the stories they tell extended family and neighbors to hide their pregnancies, of intentions that are related to material and spiritual concerns, and in terms of the view of their bodies and pregnancies as these exist between what they know and what they are being counseled to understand. For example, Durgaben, who had been through the embryo-implantation process and was waiting to find out if she was pregnant when I met her, explained how she came to be a surrogate.

> I have a friend in my neighborhood who was a surrogate [at this clinic], and she told me about this opportunity. She explained to me that my womb is like an extra room in a house that I don't need, and can be rented out. The baby stays there for nine months, so it has a place to grow, but it is not your baby.
>
> (Vora 2009, 271)

Clinic staff guide women into an understanding that the child will not have a blood relation to them because it is genetically someone else's child, primarily because its genes will not be hers. Further research needs to be done on how people who are unfamiliar with the basic biology of genetics, as is the case with the vast majority of surrogates prior to their contact with the clinic, translate and understand what they are told about genes and genetics.

The co-director of Manushi clinic, Dr. B., has explained to me and in interviews with the press that part of her job with regard to recruiting surrogates, for which she emphasizes that the clinic does not charge a fee, is that she must educate the surrogates to understand that surrogacy doesn't require sex to create a baby, as they have not before encountered technologies of IVF. This narrative, which is also recounted by surrogates, repeats the metaphors of the uterus as an empty room, and of surrogacy as letting someone else's child stay in your house for 9 months.

One of the potentializing features of gestational surrogacy that is represented in the notion of wombs for rent is a spatialization reminiscent of colonial figurations and fantasies of newly encountered land as empty and unpopulated. This figuring positions land (and resources within) as in need of organization and management to become productive, which in turn justified its seizure. Assisted reproduction, tissue engineering, and stem-cell research all share in the process of using technologies to reorganize, or reconceptualize the body, as a site of potential productivity. This creation of productivity is reproductive, speculative, and as such, valuable to the market.

The discourse of wombs for rent or in need of management also helps displace the narrative of exploitation where surrogacy is the sale of the use of one's body parts by wealthier couples, and where physicians are actually business people. It deflects the complex social friction generated by the practice of commercial surrogacy and suggests that surrogacy is simply fulfilling unrealized potential on both the side of the surrogate and of the commissioning parents. As clinic staff coach surrogates in the utility of their otherwise un-engaged uterus, and in informational literature, its website, and staff conversations with commissioning parents about the role of the surrogate as a temporary guardian of someone else's child (Vora 2014), the clinic creates a narrative of using otherwise wasted resources in the form of employing under- or unemployed Indian women as surrogates, a situation that justifies intervention and change. As an "idle machine,"[5] the womb of the would-be surrogate is abstracted from her subject and body and marked as an offense to productivity and in part justifies its own exploitation by deserving would-be parents.

Genetics is the underlying justification for the nonrelationship between surrogates and the fetuses they carry, and in everyday language surrogates utilize this discourse through referencing knowledge that the child will not look like them, though the depth of their engagement with genetic discourse is not perfectly clear. Nonetheless, I argue that the work of doctors and staff at the clinic to induct surrogates into a form of "genetic essentialism"[6] is a tool both to assure them of the moral soundness of surrogacy (it does not involve sex outside of marriage), as well as to make them understand that the baby will not be theirs, and that it is rather a foreign presence in the otherwise empty space of the uterus. As I will explain below, geneticization, the process by which genetics has come to explain health and disease, and to naturalize social differences as biologically based (Lippman 1991), is one piece of a larger project of social uplift imagined through benevolent education of surrogates by doctors, staff, and the matron of at least one of the hostels.

As mentioned above, commissioning mothers[7] are invited into the embryology lab in sterilized suits and masks to view the forming embryo under the microscope. One of the directors cited this as an example of something you could not get in a more commercial and large-scale clinic in the United States or United Kingdom, and as such was part of what made Manushi special: its attention to the clients. Also, she said, it "helps (commissioning) mothers bond with the fetus." Martin asserts that practices that push the level of analysis and observation down to the microscopic view in biology detach it from bodies and persons, and from social structures and processes, and that forcing the scale of knowledge back above the microscopic cannot undo the effects of having seen things at that level (2001, 180). The very idea that there is "something" with which to bond depends on the externalization of the fetus from the uterus, the microscope as instrument, and the visualization and discourse of the fetus. DNA explains who is supposed to bond with the cells under the microscope. As a metaphor, DNA implies a hierarchical ordering, so that the intended parents as the source of DNA (even when working with donated eggs) have more right to control the process of surrogacy than the surrogate, because the fetus is their property and she is a service provider.

The way that surrogates at Manushi clinic talk about their relationship to pregnancy and their pregnant bodies rehearses some of the clinic's metaphors, but also insists on a common sense notion that it is their body, its blood, and the food they eat and use, that is growing the infant. Surrogates explain their influence through pregnancy on the outcome of the birth. For example, one former surrogate noted that the reason her commissioning parents would have a boy is because she was very successful in producing boy children, having produced two of her own. In addition to asserting the presence of competing ideas about the nature of surrogacy (see also Pande 2009), these other modes of embodiment in surrogacy point to other possible socialities than those indicated by geneticization.

The Imagination of Debt and Future Connection

After acknowledging how difficult it was to see their husbands and children only once a week, as well as managing the isolation of living away from their homes in general, women who stayed in the hostel I visited described the positive aspect of living there throughout their pregnancy and postdelivery as an experience of sisterhood with other surrogates. Some imagined this feminine space and time away from the demands of family to be akin to staying in a student hostel, an experience most would not have had. Some women described missing others who had left after giving birth, and one woman noted that she dreaded leaving her sisters at the hostel behind after she completed her surrogacy. At the same time, many women explained that living in the hostel was a necessity because of the pressure to keep this work a secret from their extended families to escape the social stigma imposed by community members; living in the hostel gave them a place to stay away from home and out of sight. Many of the women I spoke to had told at least some neighbors and extended family, if not in-laws, that they were going to a distant city in India or as far as Dubai for a temporary job. Women whose homes were within a reasonable driving distance could entertain visits from their husbands and children on weekends, and these children were told different stories, sometimes that their mother was receiving special medical care for a health condition. In the case of one family I spoke to, the children were told that their mother was going to have a child for another family who could not have children. This desire for anonymity underlines the possible shame in this work, though surrogates emphasize that the work is morally defensible, based on the fact that the embryo is made outside the body and inserted by the doctor.[8]

Commissioning parents express a spectrum of sentiments about their future relationship to their surrogate, ranging from a vague hope that her fees will help her improve the lives of her family members, to specific goals of educating her children. These sentiments exist in the context of knowledge that given India's lack of legislation regulating surrogacy arrangements, and the social and geographical distance between their family and that of the surrogate, any future connection is ultimately entirely within their discretion. One middle-class white couple who was visiting the clinic for egg harvesting and sperm donation for IVF and surrogacy offered several reasons for choosing this clinic over a clinic in the United States, including its affordability for them after several failed IVF cycles in the United States, as well as the physical distance that would exist between their family in the United States and the clinic and their surrogate in India. Mentioning discomfort with custody claims made by former surrogates in US courts, she said, "I'm glad that she [the surrogate] will be in India and we will be in the US." The spatial imagination of distance is not only about geography, but also the implicit acknowledgment that women of the class from which surrogates are recruited, primarily women whose family members can only find casual or day labor between longer jobs doing manual and service work, will not have the education or means to track them down in the future, even if the clinic somehow failed to protect their identifying information.

Despite being told that the only relationship they will have to the intended parents of the fetus they carry to term will be transactional and temporary, discussions in the surrogacy residence hostel, and comments by aspiring and new surrogates, point to different expectations. Former surrogates I spoke with said that in spite of their coaching, they missed the children after they left India and hoped to hear about their development and to receive pictures as the child continued its life away from them. That said, none mentioned the hope of an ongoing relationship with the child specifically. For example, Sita said that she "feels good" after delivering an infant as a surrogate 1 month prior. She elaborated,

> I feel connected to that person [the commissioning mother], as if I had known this lady for a long time. She continues to call me and I feel good because she keeps calling to talk and ask how I am doing. I hope it will continue this way for my lifetime.

When directly asked about hopes for the future relation to the commissioning family, one current surrogate offered that she "would be pleased" if the child attempted to meet her after it had reached adulthood, and another surrogate mentioned that, "they [commissioning parents] should remember me on the birthday." When I asked how she should be remembered, she said, "I would want them to call," and another woman offered that, "they should send a gift on the birthday." In this way, the hope, and in some cases, attempt to create, an ongoing relationship with the commissioning parents that would continue to benefit themselves and their families in the future was first and foremost. Pande has observed this fantasy as a type of "kinship work" that Indian surrogates do in building real and fantasy ties with commissioning families across caste, class, regional and national lines (Pande 2009). Some women at Manushi described their efforts to establish a reciprocal relationship modeled on that of patron and client, rather than a claim on kinship, where the surrogate expects the commissioning parents to sustain a sense of obligation toward her after the child is given to them. Although women I spoke to admitted that it has not happened very often, there was a tendency to dwell on the stories of those rare surrogates who did receive continued or extended support or even just promises of support from their commissioning parents. In one introductory interview between a commissioning father and his assigned surrogate (since he was using donated eggs, his wife had elected not to travel to India for this first visit), she explored the extent of his intentions toward her and her family by asking if he would be willing to bring her family to the United States and help them find jobs. He did express a vague intention to help educate her children and perhaps invite them to the United States, but by the end of their contract 9 months later, he described insurmountable frustration with her continued attempts to "get more money" from him and his wife whenever they communicated. Dr. B. had earlier explained to me that part of the reason that they discourage communication between surrogates and commissioning parents, in addition to the often insurmountable language gap, was to protect commissioning parents from being pressured by the surrogates, though she said that the structure of the clinic and its surrogacy arrangements made anything like blackmail impossible.

When I spoke to women who were currently pregnant as surrogates, many described the value and meaning of surrogacy as different from a job, as apart from categories of kinship new or old, and as apart from clinic and market discourses. As was discussed in Chapter 2, there was instead an emphasis on a feeling that carrying a child for a couple that could not otherwise have a child was an extraordinary and even divine act, and that this was more important than money as a motivation (Vora 2010). Discourse about the divine aspects of surrogacy point to simultaneous and competing logics for the social meaning and value of gestational surrogacy. These meanings cannot be easily organized or communicated through the genetic definition of a biological parent, though it is a condition of possibility for commercial surrogacy, or even through the economic logic of the value of the labor of surrogacy as underpaid and technologically mediated "women's work" in the global economy.

The feeling that commissioning parents owe something to the surrogate in kind for the magnitude of the gift of a child fits into a cultural logic outlined by Jan Brouwer (1999) in her study of small business culture and its disjunctures with global business culture in India. Brouwer argues that indigenous cultural ideologies spanning India posit an economy of debt and repayment that is partially sympathetic with the economic logics of global production, but whose differences are essential. Her study of the Vishwakarma community of jewelry artisans in interior Karnataka state finds that debt and payment between goldsmiths and the commissioning businessmen who sell their work is about acknowledging the importance of open-ended social relationships.

What is read by commissioning parents as solicitation and manipulation for more money and resources by a surrogate can be seen as a way to insist on the transcendental nature of her gift, which necessarily exceeds the surrogacy fee, and creates on opening that logically insists on continuing relationality and exchange, even as it can simultaneously be a pragmatic pursuit of an opportunity for accumulating resources. This possibility of mediation that builds on indigenous and global systems simultaneously, working between the cultural logic or common sense expectations of workers and other subjects in India and the logic of neoliberal exchange and financialization, sets up an interesting context for rethinking ethics, responsibility, and regulation in transnational surrogacy, which I will take up in the last section of this essay. At the least, it creates a precedent for taking seriously the ontological and material expectations of both surrogates and commissioning parents in establishing an ethics of practice and remuneration in the clinic.

Promise and Risk

In exchange for the promise of their fee and the possible future it represents, surrogates undertake uncertainty and unknown risks in terms of their social status, their health and wellness through pregnancy and thereafter, and even the chance that they will not receive the full fee promised to them. For commissioning parents who have deferred childbearing or who have ongoing medical obstacles, the promise is that reproduction is possible. The other side of the promise of the social experiment contained in transnational Indian surrogacy, for commissioning parents and surrogates alike, is the possibility of accident or other unpredictable outcomes, and together these characterize the space of the clinic.

The promise that justifies the undertaking of risk can be as simple as the temporary end of a state of mundane crisis—the impossibility of getting by—but can also serve as a platform to imagine possible futures. For example, the sum surrogates are promised is enough to create a small platform from which it is possible to imagine another future, even if that future is simply coming closer to ends already mandated (dowry and wedding expenses, debt). On the part of surrogates, the promise also unfolds in the imagination of future assistance from commissioning parents and future employment through the clinic.

The health risks associated with pregnancy for surrogates include those inherent in all pregnancies, including, but certainly not only, complications such as preeclampsia, gestational diabetes, or problems leading to preterm birth. It is difficult to get comprehensive statistics for the nature and outcome of births associated with ART clinics in India right now because there is no required reporting (SAMA 2010). In 2008, Manushi clinic was not offering any kind of risk-related counseling to surrogates. Several surrogates volunteered that they had not had this kind of high-tech intensive prenatal care and supervision during their other pregnancies, which suggests a feeling of less risk than they faced with prior births. These would likely have been at home attended by a midwife, or for those with the means to afford it, in the local maternity hospital, but without the interventions of ultrasound or blood testing unless there was illness and money for such care. Interviews between doctors and commissioning parents I observed did not include any kind of risk counseling, though this could be the result of limited access to client interviews with doctors. The medical risks for egg donation, IVF, and surrogacy exceed even those that are routinely disclosed through contracts and counseling in more highly regulated clinics outside India, and reports from Sama—Resource Group for Women and Health (2010) indicate that there is little disclosure of risk in Indian ART clinics in general.[9] Pregnancy with multiple fetuses is common in IVF, and these pregnancies are subject to higher risks for surrogates than single pregnancies. Current draft legislation does not grant a surrogate a choice in whether or not she wishes to undergo a multiple pregnancy. Also, the hormones injected by intended mothers and surrogates alike, hormones that organize the female reproductive system to synchronize it with the clinic's schedule for egg harvest, IVF, and embryo implantation carry risks.[10]

Additional risks are posed to participants in surrogacy arrangements because of the lack of legal protection. The Indian government is excited about its position in the growth of the biotechnology industry worldwide, and as K. Sunder Rajan (2007) explains in his ethnographic work on clinical trials in India, governments must compete to attract commercial research organizations to their countries by offering laws attractive to them. Draft ART legislation in India would grant active surrogates claim to insurance through the commissioning parents "as per the agreement and till the surrogate mother is free of all health complications arising out of surrogacy" (Clause 34:23). It is difficult to imagine that someone of the social class in which most Indian surrogates find themselves would or even could pursue commissioning parents, about whom they often have very little information, for long-term health problems attributable to surrogacy such as those indicated by the recent studies mention above. The law draws out a contracted period with limited obligations to the surrogate on the part of commissioning parents, mainly the maintenance of the surrogate and mandated custody of the child once it is born "irrespective of any abnormality" (Clause 34:11). The surrogate meanwhile would be constrained by a more abstract and limiting clause, where she must not "act in any way that would harm the foetus during pregnancy and the child after birth" (Clause 34:28). The child born to a surrogate may request information about egg donors or surrogates at age 18 (Clause 36:1), as may their guardians before 18 with "prior informed consent of donor or surrogate mother." There are no equivalent rights to information for surrogates in the bill.

"Life for Life": Meaning, Politics, and Ethics of Surrogacy's Exchanges

A combination of the inability to get by, coupled with a creative imagination of possible future prosperity and reinvention through the connections and resources represented by the clinic, leads women to pursue gestational surrogacy. Echoing defenders of the market in human kidneys, Dr. B. argues that the exchange involved in surrogacy arrangements is an exchange of "life for life." This argument, equating the reproduction or preservation of life on the consuming side and the means of subsistence on the producing side, veils the differential material circumstances that make such an exchange uneven, because it implies that there is some quantum of "life itself." Examining the process by which "life itself" comes to be imagined as a unit of exchange is instructive for understanding how ARTs in the context of the Manushi clinic are not neutral instruments of human activity, but rather vehicles for the perpetuation of unequal social-material relations as well as for the invention of new ones.

Dr. B.'s promise to would-be surrogates, through a word of mouth recruiting strategy, is that she will assist them in keeping control of their earnings, even against the will of the husband and father-in-law in her house, whose money it ultimately is understood to be by the conventional patriarchal social logics of the joint family economy. Part of this project is that the husband's relationship with the clinic does not end with signing the permission form for their wives to become surrogates, but that they are also, at least by association, included in the clinic's program of uplift, or restructuring. For surrogates and sometimes their husbands, working with the clinic becomes a career plan, and this also becomes a reason that women are interested in becoming surrogates at the Manushi clinic. Former surrogates have been hired into service positions like nursing assistants or custodians, and when possible or in cases where the directors feel it will be particularly important, their husbands are also incorporated. For example, the cook in one of the hostels is the husband of a former surrogate who needed a job, as are a number of other ancillary clinic staff. The story of the husband who gave up vices like alcoholism or gambling under pressure from Dr. B. is another trope of reform or rehabilitation of husbands.

The women undertaking surrogacy describe their understanding of the risks and future potential of their work in terms that acknowledge but also exceed the clinic's discourse of surrogacy as simply the paid service of gestation and rented use of an otherwise unused uterus. Their "unreasonable" expectation of a sense of indebtedness on the part of commissioning parents could be seen as an attempt to potentialize relationships formed through the clinic and to stabilize one of the competing meanings of surrogacy as exceeding what is represented by the contract. In this sense, it could be seen as a risk-management scheme on the part of women undertaking surrogacy, and as insisting on an alternative ethics for the practice and value of gestational surrogacy. Dr. B's explanation of the clinic's project of bringing together needy surrogates and childless couples as an exchange of "life for life" is also a way of stabilizing the meaning of surrogacy, framing it in a way that recalls other commercial biological exchanges, such as the exchange of a healthy kidney for money on the part of an impoverished kidney-seller (Cohen 2003; Scheper-Hughes 2000), or the participation of an impoverished or uninsured person suffering an illness for medical treatment through clinical trial participation (Cooper 2012, 2011; Sunder Rajan 2007).

Behind the material conditions underlying the willingness of women to enter into surrogacy are structural adjustments that began in 1991 in accordance with the terms of an IMF loan to the government of India. These adjustments continue in the ongoing contraction of social welfare programs and governmental protections of the domestic economy against global free trade: the removal of farm subsidies; reductions in rural health programs; and new legislation that ignores protecting life and health (SAMA 2010) because the market will "naturally" take care of it through life-for-life exchange. The cut-backs to social welfare programs in India as well as in the nations from which commissioning parents travel falls most heavily upon those who already go about their lives in the margins of society's sphere of wealth and power, where more and more women cannot conceive without assistance, largely due to preventable secondary causes like malnutrition and unsafe routine gynecological surgeries (Inhorn 2003, 1840). Instead, these cases of infertility are cited as justification for the expansion and protection of technological intervention, creating a situation where fewer and fewer people have the option of procreation without the intervention of biomedicine. "Life for life" materializes a dependent and arguably colonizing relation, justifying the conditions that lead subjects into ultimately unequal exchanges. Ironically, as K. Sunder Rajan (2007, 76) explains, the uncoupling of therapeutic access and experimental subjectivity means that experimental subjects like those participating in clinical trials in India, and I would add surrogates participating in commercial surrogacy to a lesser extent, contribute to an abstract idea of "health" as a social good, but have no access to the results in terms of their individual health.[11]

In a 2009 report, Sama—Resource Group for Women and Health indicated that people from all parts of society in India are seeking ART treatments, though they are primarily accessed by middle and upper classes. The growth of the Indian middle class has been a precondition and indeed creates the conditions of possibility for the growth of commercial surrogacy in India, along with the success of some sectors of India's diaspora who have returned to India for reproductive health care. A lifestyle change where young families choose career advancement over procreation, the structural adjustments in governmental economic policies which favor the growth of the transnational capitalist class over the ever-growing numbers of those who earn less, and the cultural imperative to become a subject of consumption (Vora, 2014) set the stage for the success of the transnational ART clinic, as well as the continued growth of the surrogacy industry. In light of this possible and even likely future, it will remain essential to ensure rights that allow participants to control the risk they face through the intervention of the state legal apparatus. Such rights might include the right to elect whether or not to undergo a multiple pregnancy, which at this moment is not in their realm of choice, despite it increasing their risk, and the right to arrange an open surrogacy and therefore future connection to the commissioning family; these are rights that are not supported by the ART bill in its current form. Feminist activists also advocate for media literacy training for future surrogates, donors and parents, rather than just reform of the problematic informed consent apparatus (SAMA 2010).

Conclusion

Dwelling on the tensions and dynamics that arise between doctors, commissioning parents, surrogates, and other actors in the clinic highlights how ART clinics, along with global inequality, simultaneously potentialize bodies and social relations in unequal forms of exchange. The unregulated nature of ART clinics in India potentializes the bodies of Indian women who need financial resources as having reproductive capacity that can benefit others. This reproductive capacity benefits the commissioning parents, who receive a child in exchange for a fee that is very low for the international market. It also benefits the doctors and the brokers who connect doctors and patients, who reap profits by manipulating the vast difference in earning between surrogates and commissioning parents. This potentializing of bodies entails risks for participants, and particularly surrogates, who risk their health, the stability of their families, and their reputations. The potentializing of social relations engendered through surrogacy arrangements allows commissioning parents to pursue a biological child through a form of surrogacy promoted as improving the conditions of women who act as surrogates, while creating opportunities for surrogates to attempt to establish extra-contractual connections to commissioning parents, the clinic, and other surrogates as a way to create future opportunities and resources for their families. It leads the clinic, including physicians and staff, to portray itself to both surrogates and commissioning parents as an entry point for women, through education and property ownership, into India's seemingly endless promise of economic growth, while building the foundation for a financially lucrative transnational medical practice.

Notes

1 When women are pressured or required to leave their homes to live in designated surrogate housing during pregnancy as surrogates, a structural situation is created that parallels what Colen (1995) has called "stratified reproduction" and that Parreñas (2000) has called the "international transfer of caretaking" (569) in the context of transnational care and domestic labor migration, where women leave their children to invest that care work into the households of families with greater financial resources.

2 This excerpt is from field notes describing events on January 29, 2008.

3 Dr. H. described this process as the fertilization, culturing and transfer of a single egg and embryo, though in reality several embryos and occasionally more will be transferred, depending on how doctors calculate the likelihood of successful pregnancy.

4 See for example: Ali and Kelly 2008; " 'Wombs for rent' grows in India."

5 Emily Martin tracks the historical "horror" at lack of productivity among capitalist subjects in the global north, citing "the factory, the failed business, the idle machine" (2001, 45).

6 Sarah Franklin describes genetic essentialism as "a scientific discourse . . . with the potential to establish social categories based on an essential truth about the

body (Franklin, 1993, 34; cited in Haraway 1997, 147). Martin (1990:153) cites Latour (2001): "the essential features of modern power: change of scale and displacement through workshop and laboratories." In this change of scale, something very minute, discovered by science, comes to play a deciding role in human questions or concerns that are very large" (171).

7 I did not hear of any fathers, though I can imagine that they would be invited in the absence of a mother.

8 A position supported by Pande's (2009) and Saravanan's (2010) studies.

9 SAMA—Resource Group for Women and Health is a non-governmental organization based in New Delhi, India, www.samawomenshealth.org/

10 For example, Lupron (leuprolide acetate) is the drug used (off-label) most often to shut down ovaries before they are stimulated with other drugs to produce multiple follicles for egg harvesting in preparation for IVF and for egg donation. There have been no long term studies of Lupron exist, but a long list of side-effects have been reported to the FDA. Studies also indicate a statistically significant higher risk of ovarian tumors among IVF patients, as well as ovarian hyperstimulation syndrome (SAMA 2010, 95). See also Lowry, 2012.

11 Sunder Rajan notes that in some rare instances, a particular trial-sponsoring company may elect to offer therapies to trial subjects through so-called "compassionate use" programs (2007, 76).

Works Cited

Ali, Loraine and Raina Kelly. (2008). "The Curious Lives of Surrogates," *Newsweek*, March 29.

American Public Media. (2007). "'Wombs for Rent' Grows in India," *Marketplace*, December 27. www.marketplace.org/topics/life/wombs-rent-grows-india.

Brouwer, Jan. (1999). "Modern and Indigenous Perceptions in Small Enterprises," *Economic and Political Weekly*, 34(48): 52–156.

Cohen, Lawrence. (2003). "Where It Hurts: Indian Material for an Ethics of organ Transplantation," *Zygon*, 38(3): 663–688.

Colen, S. (1995). "'Like a Mother to Them': Stratified Reproduction and West Indian Childcare Workers and Employers in New York," in *Conceiving the New World Order: The Global Politics of Reproduction*, Faye Ginsburg and Rayna Rapp, eds. Berkeley: University of California Press, pp. 78–102.

Cooper, Melinda. (2011). "Trial by Accident: Experiment and the Production of Surplus," paper presented at the Modern Language Association Annual Meeting, Los Angeles, January 7.

Cooper, Melinda. (2012). "The Pharmacology of Distributed Experiment: User-Generated Drug Innovation," *Body and Society*, 18(3–4): 18–43.

Franklin, Sarah. (1993). "Essentialism, Which Essentialism? Some Implications of Reproductive and Genetic Techno-Science," *Journal of Homosexuality*, 24(3–4): 27–40.

Haraway, Donna J. (1997). *Modest_Witness@Second_Millennium.FemaleMan__Meets_OncoMouse_: Feminism and Technoscience*. New York: Routledge.

Inhorn, M.C. (2003). "Global Infertility and the Globalization of New Reproductive Technologies: Illustrations from Egypt," *Social Science and Medicine*, 56(9): 1837–1851.

Latour, Bruno. (2001). "Postmodern? No, Simply Amodern! Steps Towards an Anthropology of Science," *Studies in the History and Philosophy of Science*, 21(1): 145–171.

Lippman, Abby. (1991). "Prenatal Genetic Testing and Screening: Constructing Needs and Reinforcing Inequalities," *American Journal of Law and Medicine*, 17(1–2): 15–50.

Lowry, Fran. (2012). "IVF Linked to Increased Risk for Birth Defects: Study," *Modern Medicine*, October 23. www.modernmedicine.com/news/ivf-linked-increased-risk-birth-defects-study.

Martin, Emily. (1990). *Flexible Bodies*. Boston, MA: Beacon Press.

Martin, Emily. (2001). *The Woman in the Body: A Cultural Analysis of Reproduction*. Boston, MA: Beacon Press.

Pande, Amrita. (2009). "It May Be Her Eggs but It Is My Blood: Surrogates and Everyday Forms of Kinship in India," *Qualitative Sociology*, 32(4): 379–397.

Parreñas, Rhacel Salazar. (2000). "Migrant Filipina Domestic Workers and the International Division of Reproductive Labor," *Gender and Society*, 14(4): 560–580.

Pritchard, Jack A. and Paul C. MacDonald. (1985). *Williams Obstetrics*, 17th edition. Norwalk, CT: Appleton-Century-Crofts.

SAMA Resource Group for Women and Health. (2010). *Unraveling the Fertility Industry: Challenges and Strategies for Movement Building*. New Delhi: International Consultation on Commercial, Economic, and Ethical Aspects of Assisted Reproductive Technologies. www.samawomenshealth.org/downloads/Final%20 Consultation%20Report.pdf.

Saravanan, Sheela. (2010). "European Conference on Modern South Asian Studies," conference proceedings, Bonn, Germany, July.

Scheper-Hughes, Nancy. (2000). "The Global Traffic in Human Organs," *Current Anthropology*, 41(2): 191–224.

Simpson, Bob. (2013). "Managing Potential in Assisted Reproductive Technologies: Reflections on Gifts, Kinship, and the Process of Vernacularization," *Current Anthropology*, 54(suppl. 7): S87–S96.

Sunder Rajan, Kaushik. (2007). "Experimental Values: Indian Clinical Trials and Surplus Health," *New Left Review*, 45: 67–88.

Taussig, Karen-Sue, Klaus Hoeyer and Stefan Helmreich. (2013). "The Anthropology of Potentiality in Biomedicine: An Introduction to Supplement 7," *Current Anthropology*, 54(suppl. 7): S3–S14, October.

Vora, Kalindi. (2009). "Indian Transnational Surrogacy and the Commodification of Vital Energy," *Subjectivities*, 28(1): 266–278.

Vora, Kalindi. (2010). "Medicine, Markets and the Pregnant Body: Indian Commercial Surrogacy and Reproductive Labor in a Transnational Frame," *Scholar and Feminist Online*, 9(1–2). http://sfonline.barnard.edu/reprotech/vora_01.htm.

Vora, Kalindi. (2014). "Experimental Socialities and Gestational Surrogacy in the Indian ART Clinic," *Ethnos: Journal of Anthropology*, 79(1): 63–83.

7

EXPERIMENTAL SOCIALITY IN TRANSNATIONAL SURROGACY

In addition to being a site of producing women's bodies in particular, and contracted reproduction in general, as sites of potentiality the transnational surrogacy clinic and the contractual relations it fosters result in experimental forms of sociality among participants. In the early days of commercial surrogacy in India, the improvised nature of what was a new and novel form of medical service meant that the clinic acted as a contact zone for the elite doctors, gestational surrogates, and transnational commissioning parents convening there. This essay examines efforts within one assisted reproductive technology (ART) clinic to separate social relationships from reproductive bodies in its surrogacy arrangements and the improvised social formations the formed both because of and despite of these efforts.[1] These social formations emerge as experiments with different forms of modernity in the space of the clinic. These experiments include occupying different relationships to physical bodies and the social meaning of medicalized biological reproduction, underlined as these are by a variety of understandings of the role of both the market and of altruism in the practice of gestational surrogacy.

This essay draws on observations and interviews conducted in 2008 in Northern India as well as follow-up interviews with doctors and commissioning parents through 2016. It examines some of the ways that participants negotiate the meaning of surrogacy arrangements through experimental modes of sociality, both in practice and imagination, in the context of the clinic. As a contact zone, the clinic is an unusual social space in that is brings together middle-class but demographically elite doctors, elite Indian commissioning parents, nonresident Indian and transnational commissioning parents,[2] and rural women who wish to become surrogates and have comparatively few resources, including finances, education, connections, and governmental investment. Here, they are meeting and inter-relating in addition to exchanging money and services. In the tradition of medical anthropology, I observed these interactions and practices as constituting an important site of social analysis in themselves, rather than intending to make claims about individuals' social worlds outside the clinic. For broader

 DOI: 10.4324/9781003353362-7

context, this essay also references legislation around ARTs in India, and draws upon longer-term observation of the rise of other globally oriented and technology-based industries in India through fieldwork conducted intermittently between 2004 and 2006.

The transnational market in surrogacy renders the Manushi clinic as a space of mediated social interaction that shapes the ways that doctors, commissioning parents, and surrogates can interact. The space of the clinic is already defined at least in part through the relationship of exchange bringing together participants. This relationship gets materialized through the surrogacy contract and the intervention of medical technologies and knowledge that makes gestational surrogacy possible. These market-enabled conditions in turn impact the way that people understand their bodies and their modes of engagement in relation to one another. As a result, we can see modes of social experimentation emerge "as a subjective orientation towards the world and towards society, moving [experimentation] beyond the realm of medical anthropology into the larger field of material culture and consumption as these are characterized by a mode of inhabiting rapidly shifting and increasingly global social/market contact zones" (Towghi and Vora 2014). Experimentation with different modes of being and subjective orientations to the world has become central to the very meaning of what it means to be modern (Ibid.) One place in which such experimentation happens is in the ways that surrogates and commissioning parents navigate around structures and practices in the clinic designed to separate social relationships from reproductive bodies. Experimental social relations occur in the imagination of participants as they consider what their future relationship might be despite being discouraged to communicate by doctors and staff. Another place in which efforts to establish experimental socialities occurs is in the connections that form between commissioning parents and surrogates despite efforts to contain them. Other experimental socialities form as a direct result of how the clinic has structured its medical practice, such as those between commissioning parents as they share information and anxieties about medical and legal details of contracting a surrogate or of navigating medical travel in India. Also, though relationships between surrogates living in the clinics residence hostels are not at the heart of the clinic's intended goals for surrogacy, they support its success while also providing opportunities for conversation and collaboration between women residing there. Through the lens of medical anthropology and the history of medicine, these experiments in sociality can be understood to reflect a shift in medicine away from a technique of caring for the body, or pastoral care, to one of producing bodies as the instruments of service work and surrogates as entrepreneurs of the contracted use of those instruments.[3] This analysis is supported by language in the several drafts of legislation proposed to regulate commercial surrogacy in India between 2008 and 2016, and entails an uneven distribution of risk among participants in gestational surrogacy that has become an issue of national debate as well as impacting the way that participants imagine their relationships to one another through surrogacy arrangements and beyond.

Background

The Manushi clinic is located in a modest building within a hospital complex found in the center of a small city in northwestern India. It is difficult to find without local advice. The clinic itself consists of a large waiting room in which there is a freestanding registration desk and an adjacent restroom, three examination rooms along a hallway that is separated from the waiting room by a fabric curtain, a nurses' station, and two office suites for the co-directors of the clinic. Dr. T,[4] one of the clinic's co-directors, meets visitors in one of these offices. It serves as the de facto public relations office, and as the reception and waiting area for wealthy Indian and foreign visitors, clients, and patients of the clinic. With cushioned conference-style chairs arranged around Dr. T's large desk, and a recently renovated restroom with a western style toilet, this office offers a more familiar and comfortable experience for these client-patients than the public waiting area. It also illustrates the juxtaposition of a newer, private style of medicine offered by the clinic with the larger-scaled public medicine represented by the older waiting room. There local patients of the general OB/GYN practice that operates as part of the hospital's general services leave their shoes outside, and after entering, sit in plastic chairs fully lining each wall.

The clinic's transnational practice began when nonresident Indians, home to visit family in the area, began to seek treatment for reproductive ailments from the highly trained Dr. B. Already performing in vitro fertilization (IVF) and laparoscopic reproductive surgeries with great success and for prices that were far lower than those in their home countries, in the early 2000s Dr. B agreed to a request by a former patient to attempt gestational surrogacy. This patient had arranged for a family member to act as her gestational carrier. The case was a success, and through word of mouth and newspaper articles in the United Kingdom and India, the surrogacy practice began to grow. A decade later, the clinic receives as many as 10,000 emails regarding their gestational surrogacy practice per month, and though it is a very small clinic, it hired a full-time staff person just to manage correspondence generated by press coverage and visitors to its web site. In 2008, there were an average of 50 active gestational carrier pregnancies at a given time, the maximum the clinic could support in terms of its personnel and housing resources. The clinic directors emphasized that women interested in becoming surrogates came after hearing about them through word of mouth, and were strictly self-referred, a significant difference from other clinics who rely on brokers to recruit surrogates. The clinic attributes their successful word-of-mouth recruiting to the efforts it has made to teaching women to invest their surrogacy fees in newly constructed homes, education, and setting up small businesses. The wait list for people meeting the initial criteria for eligibility for gestational surrogacy has as many as 500 entries.

A set of cottage industries has grown around the new traffic to the clinic, forming something like a small tourism industry. Foreign clients arrive to the clinic in different ways, but for most, Dr. T arranges in advance for one of two drivers employed by the clinic, a set of brothers connected to clinic staff, to meet them at the airport. At the patient's expense, one of the brothers makes the trip of over an hour to the nearest airport to bring newly arrived patients to town. Many foreign clients described later choosing to hire one of the drivers to give them tours and to take them on day-trips out of town during their visit to the clinic, a practice promoted by Dr. T. Clients are set up to stay in the local hotel, nice by local standards but not qualifying for the international hotel star ratings system, also by Dr. T's staff. At the time of my visit, plans for building an internationally rated hotel for foreign patients were being discussed, gesturing to the clinic's interest in expanding its hospitality interests, through the directors emphasized their disinterest in being a business, instead described the hotel plan as a way to make foreign guests more comfortable during their visits.

Commissioning Parents

During the day, Dr. T's office serves as a check in point for foreign commissioning parents, who pass in and out as they wait for various tests or procedures at the clinic. During my visit, one couple that frequented this room were Reeta and Sanjay, British Indian parents whose surrogate had borne twins just 1 week earlier. They were now waiting for the mandated 3-month period required by British law before bringing home a child born abroad through surrogacy. Their twins were born early and underweight, through cesarian section, and were housed in the neonatal intensive care unit (NICU) where they would stay until they reached the required weight. When visiting hours in the NICU ended, or when their surrogate arrived to breastfeed the infants, the couple would stop into the office. This surrogate, whom I never had the opportunity to meet, was a Hindu woman from a town near the clinic, and was reportedly recovering without incident. Though clinic directors told me that surrogates usually only breastfeed newborn infants for 2 or 3 days after delivery to give them some immune benefits, anecdotal evidence suggested that a number of recently delivered and former surrogates were currently or had in the past been breastfeeding infants for 2 weeks to 3 months after delivery.

New arrivals to Dr. T's office were offered no entertainment while waiting other than conversation. Reeta, the new mother, described to a rapt and often emotional group of commissioning parents how she had spent large periods of time over the last 20 years trying to become a mother, first through hormonal fertility therapies and then primarily through IVF. Other commissioning parents were eager to hear these stories which suggested their own possible success in having a child. Reeta mentioned that at several times over the years she and her husband Sanjay had considered adoption. However, in the end they decided that it was essential that their child be Indian and vegetarian from conception. They first heard about surrogacy in India when Dr. B. gave a lecture on her work at the Manushi clinic to their local chapter of the Vishwa Hindu Parishad, an international Hindu diaspora organization. At the time, she was traveling on a speaking tour of Indian immigrant communities in the United Kingdom. She described how they realized that this was the perfect opportunity to finally have a child that fit their ideals in terms of both its shared genetics and through the nature of the gestational carrier's body/womb ("vegetarian"). She said that the clinic offered them use of its human ova bank, where all donors are local Indian women, and an Indian gestational surrogate.

In talking about their efforts to have children over the last 20 years, Sanjay expressed frustration with what he described as the limitations of the British legal system. In the United Kingdom, commercial surrogacy arrangements are not legal, and surrogacy is only allowed as an altruistic act. Commissioning parents from other countries with similar legal limits on commercial surrogacy arrangements also discuss these as central to the decision to pursue surrogacy in India rather than at home. These legal limitations can include limits on the number of embryos allowed for implantation (an indicator of the likely success of a given IVF cycle or gestational surrogacy attempt), laws about when infants born through surrogacy abroad may be repatriated, and laws concerning the stance of public or private medical institutions toward financial coverage of fertility technologies. Sanjay described periods of depression Reeta suffered in alternation with feelings of desperation and determination to conceive a child. He described her how her career success as a manager in a financial institution and other stability in her life was not enough. She could not be happy until she had a child. As high-caste Gujarati Hindus living abroad who clearly maintained an investment in Gujarati Brahmin notions of vegetarianism and bodily/spiritual/caste purity around diet, Reeta and Sanjay found in the Manushi clinic an opportunity to both skirt British laws governing surrogacy and insure the conventions of Gujarati Brahmin vegetarianism from the moment of conception.

Another couple that frequented the office and was part of group conversations with Reeta and Sanjay was Karen, a homemaker, and her husband Jim, a salesman from the United States. Karen explained how more than 3 years of failed IVF cycles in the United States lead to feelings of alienation and hopelessness. She described how clinic staff in the United States referred to her exclusively by her patient number, and of having no consistent relationship with any given clinician. She contrasted this to 10 days that she had spent at the Manushi clinic, where she felt and also received very personalized attention and care. Their reasons for coming to India were primarily cost-based, though Karen added that they had shopped around, looking into a few other fertility clinics offering gestational surrogacy in India before finally choosing Manushi:

> [The other clinics] felt like such a business. I mean obviously everyone does things for financial gain, but it just had a very negative feel to it, and being here it feels like you are helping someone who really needs it and they are doing something amazing for you. It is such a positive feeling for you. This clinic seemed much more open and like they weren't hiding anything.

Karen's comment about "helping someone" references the clinic's discursive emphasis on assisting women who become gestational surrogates, primarily by managing their surrogacy fees in a way the clinic believes will have lasting material impact. A number of foreign (non-Indian) commissioning parents expressed similar sentiments. They described feeling that the relatively high fees the clinic claimed to pay these rurally based Indian women (roughly $7000—equivalent to 8 or 9 years of regular income), in conjunction with the clinic's emphasis on the social work imperative of the clinic, mitigated their own potential role in exploiting gestational surrogates through fee-based surrogacy arrangements.

The clinic's messaging around its informal program of uplift for surrogates is that it strongly encourages women who have been surrogates to manage their finances in highly specific ways. In January 2008, the clinic directors had begun to offer to place the fees earned by surrogates into trust accounts so that the money could be preserved, upon the woman's request, until the time was right to use it for the purpose she wished. When she requests the funds be released from the trust, the clinic would directly pay a home-builder, bank trust, or other approved purposes. Clinic staff described how in the past women would "misuse" their fees, choosing (with the influence of husband and in-laws) to buy cars, scooters, or other consumables, and in at least one anecdote, the money was spent on a husband's gambling habit. Another popular use for surrogacy earnings had been to fund large-scale religious ceremonies and rituals. Though such ceremonies could be interpreted as redistributing wealth gained through surrogacy in the immediate community, the directors saw all of these uses as wasteful. They began casually counseling the surrogates on how to use their earnings to buy a house, start a business, or fund the future education of their children. These were the only uses for surrogacy fees that were given to me by clinic staff members, though a number of surrogates talked about paying off debt or saving for dowries additional goals. As mentioned above, these stories aid in recruiting potential surrogates as well as creating a platform for commissioning parents to imagine a form of benevolent, distant, and continued social impact and relatedness to surrogates' lives through the fees they pay for surrogacy.

ARTs, Embodiment, and Experimental Socialities

Due to the clinic's policy that a commissioning mother have proven medical need of a gestational surrogate, many couples require donor ova. Dr. B. described the clinic process for matching egg donors and commissioning parents as fully anonymous on both sides, which is also how she describes matching gestational surrogate candidates with commissioning parents. In both cases, clinic directors personally make these selections. Anecdotal evidence, such as Sanjay and Reeta's story, where parents have specific needs or requests (here a vegetarian surrogate, potentially code for caste Brahmin), suggest that these protocols are not always rigidly followed. Dr. T described the clinic's psychological screening practice for women interested in becoming surrogates as similarly personal and casual. He said he himself interviews candidates, and that "you know if they are the right type. You get a sense right away if this person is serious." These selection practices form part of Dr. B's emphasis on the clinic's refusal to engage in what she describes as making designer-babies. This emphasis also carries into her insistence that the clinic only accepts commissioning (heterosexual) couples where the intended mother cannot successfully carry a pregnancy on her own (usually because of uterine complications or sustained failure of embryo-attachment in the uterus). Though they did not advertise it and in fact avoided discussing it, the clinic occasionally would accept individual men as clients intending to have a child using a donor egg and a gestational surrogate. The clinic publicly advertises that it does not contract with same-sex couples, however, they do accept single-parent clients which represent an opportunity for one partner in a same-sex household to apply. The additional criteria for intending parents who wish to have a child through gestational surrogacy using their own gametes is that they have blood work done to make sure that they are healthy enough for sperm and egg donation. Women must provide evidence that they are unable to carry a pregnancy on their own. For women interested in becoming gestational, the clinic requires blood work that clears them of any possible chronic medical conditions or illnesses. The husbands of women interested in becoming surrogates must also undergo bloodwork to test for any diseases that could transmit to their wives. The clinic requires any candidate for becoming a gestational surrogate to already have given birth to at least one child, to be married, and to be under the age of 40. All of these requirements were individually designed by this clinic with consideration to safety, practicality, and marketability, as India had not passed legislation to govern ART practice as of March 2012.

In describing the things that set it apart from ART and surrogacy clinics in the United States and the United Kingdom, the Manushi clinic emphasizes the high-tech aspects of its services. Pre-implantation embryo viewing and four-dimensional (4D) ultrasound, processes that may not be available to patients elsewhere, are emphasized by directors to clients, the press, on the clinic website, and in their correspondence and communication with prospective clients. The staff embryologist at the clinic told me that she knew of no other clinic that invited intended mothers into the embryology lab to view embryos under the microscope before implantation (there was no mention of inviting intended fathers during my period of observation). Dr. T described this as a way to encourage the intended mother to feel she was centrally involved in the pregnancy despite the fact that most commissioning parents leave India after initial testing and the collection of gametes for IVF. If they are present before the surrogate's delivery, intended parents are also invited to attend a 4D sonography session in the late stages of the surrogate's pregnancy. Women who had been or currently were working as surrogates did not mention their experiences or interpretation of these ultrasound sessions to me. However, based on the many rigorous studies of similar uses of visualizing technologies (Rapp 1999; Martin 2001; Stabile 1998), this use of visualizing technology to create intimacy and sociality between the commissioning parents and the fetus can be assumed to simultaneously erase the woman acting as a gestational surrogate, at least in the perception of the commissioning parents. Current and former surrogates at this clinic noted that they had not had prior exposure to technologically mediated care in pregnancies with their own children (Vora 2011, 2015). The clinic's promotional emphasis on their use of cutting edge technologies, together with promotion of Dr. B's high level of specialty obstetrics training in India and abroad, fits the general pattern of how medical treatment and services by Indian hospitals, facilitators, and brokers are marketed to foreigners, as does the emergence of cottage tourist industries for travel and tourism around medical services (Crooks et al. 2011, 5). As insurance plans in countries with privately funded medical programs adjust their requirements to accommodate the lower-priced treatments and therapies available internationally, the discourse surrounding the marketing of medical travel will likely adjust as well.

As observed in the way that its uses medical visualizing technologies, the Manushi clinic makes efforts to separate participants and potential social relations from the components of conception and gestation that will eventually produce a child for the intended parents. Staff contribute in their communication with potential and active surrogates and commissioning parents by emphasizing IVF technology as depersonalizing the components of reproduction. Administrative and technical staff generally described the process of gestational surrogacy as yielding only one set of parents. The surrogate in turn is described as performing a role that is altruistic yet ultimately a service. Even so, some participants continued to attach physical and cultural traits to the process of surrogacy, even in subtle ways. For instance in the account of Reeta and Sanjay, the British nonresident Indian (NRI) couple described above, who described the priority to hire a gestation surrogate whose personal choices were in keeping with their embodied standards of race/ethnicity and caste and/or religious purity ("vegetarian"). Despite these discursive efforts, actual individualized bodies and the relations they entail lingered in clinic interactions. In another example, administrative staff mentioned in passing several of the egg donors used at the clinic were employed as custodial and nursing staff when they were recruited. Though the clinic protocol for matching egg donors and intended parents was described by directors as their personal matching of fully anonymous egg-donors and intended parents,[5] one staff person told me unofficially that the directors choose egg donors with "light skin and eyes" for foreign commissioning parents. At the same time, I was assured by Dr. T. that foreign clients did not concern themselves with the caste of the egg-donor. In general, the clinic directors deferred questions about how they made decisions about matching egg donors and commissioning parents. As a result, they offered no other specific information about the physical characteristics or caste backgrounds of egg donors.

From the beginning of recruitment of surrogates and through the process of surrogacy, the medical and upper administrative staff of the clinic worked to distance them from intended parents. These efforts occurred alongside the self-conscious attempts by clinic staff to train surrogates to think of their bodies through a western medical lens. Doctors and staff upheld the narrative that they must explain to women interested in becoming surrogates how surrogacy works in a very rudimentary way, because most women have not had the level of formal education that would expose them to the basics of in vitro fertilization. Doctors and staff also described these explanations as essential to assure potential surrogates that there is nothing sexual involved in surrogacy. In addition, this coaching served to direct surrogates toward the desired understanding that they would have a distanced relationship to the infant they would gestate and deliver. Potential surrogates were coached to understand their uterus as an empty space they could loan to a childless couple, a place for that couple's child to stay temporarily. Most importantly, they were coached to understand that because the infant they would bear would not be a part of their life and would not resemble them physically. This fetus and eventual infant would by the beneficiary of their body's space (the uterus) and service (care around the pregnancy).

The clinic staff's instrumentalized medical description to potential and active surrogates of how reproductive technologies work encourages distance between participants and their embodiment of human reproduction. It creates a framework for commissioning parents, doctors, and surrogates to imagine the act of gestating a child as a paid occupation, where a service (gestation and childbirth) is exchanged for a fee. This does not mean that the exchange is actually delimited by these terms. Rather, medical discourse isolates the reproductive body and gametes from the social context in which they originated in a way that makes women "free" to sell gestation and childbirth as services to commissioning parents who are "free" to hire these services from a woman as labor. Without the alienating discourse of medical science and reproductive technology, the nature of gestation and childbirth would remain tied to bodies and sex for women working as surrogates, just as it continues to be among those in their home communities. It could also potentially be more difficult for commissioning parents to understand their relationship to the surrogate as ending with delivery, and to understand the surrogate as anonymous in terms of shaping the biology and personhood of the infant. In these ways, biogenetic explanations of kinship and the separation of bodies from social reproduction in the clinic participate in the experimental production of surrogates as a type of laboring subject rather than strictly a subject of kinship or of altruistic giving (as is ostensibly the case in countries like the United Kingdom where it is illegal to arrange a surrogacy outside of an altruistic agreement).

Market logics, which structure access to gametes, women willing to enter gestational surrogacy contracts, and the technologies of assisted reproduction work alongside medico-genetic discourse to alienate the role of participants in human reproduction from social relations. These logics work efficiently with the current legal status of the ART clinic in India as private enterprise largely outside of government regulation. However, as I will explain below, clinics are still highly surveilled and informally regulated. Experimental forms of sociality arise both as a result of specifics regulations, such as in the anonymity and social separation between the genetic progenitors and parents of a child born through gestational surrogacy, as well as in addition to it, or even despite it, as in the example of relationships formed in the hostels where surrogates are more or less required to live during their pregnancies.

Experimenting with Socialities in the Surrogate Hostel

Several forms of sociality formed around, and despite, the clinic's attempt to maintain what they saw as a desirable distance between actors in the clinic. One was a system of support and feeling of kinship between surrogates. The clinic strongly encouraged gestational surrogates to live in one of several hostels they maintain for surrogates near the clinic. These were explained by staff as demonstrating commitment and responsibility for the well-being of women acting as surrogates (Vora 2009, 2011). Their room and board was paid for by the commissioning parents and the hostels were promoted to both potential clients and to potential surrogates as a way to spare women the work of caring for their own families or doing typically manual waged-work while pregnant. Hostels were also described as places where nutritious meals prepared by hired cooks and access to medical care was always available. The practice of providing housing to surrogates also served to control variables of behaviors and exposure that are understood to potentially endanger the fetus or the surrogate's health while pregnant, and more generally to provide peace of mind to commissioning parents. In the clinic's narrative, hostels provided peach of mind also to the surrogates themselves.

Women I spoke to who had or were currently staying in the hostel described the main benefit of living there throughout their pregnancy and post-delivery as an experience of sisterhood with other surrogates. This was despite rivalries and disputes. After acknowledging how difficult it was to see their husbands and children only once a week, as well as to manage the isolation of living away from their homes in general, The vast majority of current and former surrogates, and all of those I spoke with, had not had the opportunity to attend college, and some described imagining their experience away from the demands of family in this feminine space to be analogous to living in a student dormitory or hostel. Some women described missing others who had left after they had given birth, and one woman noted that she dreaded the time when she would leave her sisters at the hostel behind after she completed her surrogacy. At the same time, many women explained that there is also a pressing need to keep this work a secret from their extended families to escape social stigma imposed by community members, and so living in the hostel is a necessary separation from home and therefore an undesirable measure. This need for anonymity underlines the potential for shame in this work, though surrogates emphasize that the work is in fact morally defensible, which Amrita Pande's study of commercial Indian surrogacy also reflects (Pande 2009b). Case studies by Sheela Saravanan of four Indian women who were gestational surrogates in a similar clinic in 2009 suggests that there are also power struggles in such hostels that make some women's lives there tense or unhappy. Her case studies also assert that the grief of giving the infant to its intended parents can be extensive (Saravanan 2010). In a related discussion of the impact of postmodern and neoliberal global political and economic restructuring in the Philippines and on the concomitant formation of political subjects and projects, Neferti Tadiar insists that,

> In the midst of the [increasing reliance] on service labor and the social logics of cooperation invented by the private sector . . . these practices of care are fundamental because they create and sustain the subjective conditions of that labor . . . At the same time, these practices of experience are tangential to [those strategies].
>
> (Tadiar 2009, 260)

Tadiar's observation of the social logics and "practices of care" that evolve out of service labor organized by private interests both supports those interests as well as being tangential to them. The bonds that form between women living in the hostel as the result of their shared conditions, their sisterhood, work simultaneously to keep them in the hostels where the clinic wants them to reside for purposes of surveillance, hence making the clinic more attractive to potential commissioning parents, while also creating new relationships between women acting as surrogates and discourse about the meaning and value of surrogacy outside the discourses of the market and the clinic.

Current surrogates also described the expectation of a sustained sense of obligation on the part of commissioning parents toward themselves and their families, a form of work Pande describes as fantasy "kinship work" to build ties with commissioning families across caste, class, regional, and national lines (Pande 2009a). Women living in the hostel for active surrogates related stories of former surrogates who had continued contact with commissioning parents as a model for what they hoped would come in the future from their surrogacy arrangements, even while acknowledging that not many surrogates have established extended relationships beyond a few initial phone calls after commissioning parents return home. Commissioning parents instead experimented with notions of rehabilitation and development of the job opportunities and material conditions of surrogates by imagining the ways they might use their fees to improve their lives. Several current surrogates described an expectation that commissioning parents would naturally feel a sense of duty toward her and her household following the delivery of their child. Even though no one expressed a sense of expected kinship with the future child resulting from the surrogacy agreement, they experimented with ways that a South Asian model of the duty of a patron towards a client could play out. In these imagined scenarios commissioning parents might maintain communication and send gifts or money to support her and her family through the development of their child, such as remembering her at birth anniversaries, or make a larger investment through helping with the education of her own children.

While surrogates and commissioning parents alike experimented with fantasies of how their connection might or might not play out into the imagined future, in contrast to the open-ended future described by surrogates, commissioning parents spoke of the distance they imagined would always separate their surrogate from their family as part of the appeal of pursuing surrogacy in India. The future scenarios they described experimented with the social meaning of the excess gift nature of surrogacy by imagining fees as contributing to a project of uplift to be managed by the clinic in the future and accomplished through the same fees, and as such not entailing an extended interpersonal relationship between themselves and their surrogate. All of these imagined forms of reciprocity can be understood as experimentation with the forms of sociality that might result from the obligation and creation of a relationship through the Maussian gift nature of surrogacy, which exceeds its contractual and fee-based nature as emphasized by the clinic, together with the entanglement of bodies and novel social contexts arising with ARTS and transnational surrogacy arrangements.

Discussion: Risk, Structural Inequality, and ART legislation

In debates about the regulation of commercial surrogacy in India raised by the ART bill first drafted in 2008, but still not passed into law, lawyers, scholars, activists, and the popular press have raised questions about the risk surrounding various participants, including egg donors, surrogates, commissioning parents, and the individuals born through surrogacy. The newness of the transnational service market in ARTs in India and the government's continuing hesitance to make hard laws rather than just guidelines to govern medical and commercial practices in ART clinics, and the corresponding lack of precedents on both the levels of national and international law, as exemplified by the "Baby Manji" case, raise questions about the risk surrounding various participants.[6] Subjects facing the risks associated with the unpredictable social, legal, and medical risks arising with the development of this industry include egg donors, surrogates, commissioning parents, and the individuals born through surrogacy. The safety of egg donors as medical subjects as well as their informed consent may not be guaranteed. The surrogate undergoes risks as both an individual subject and as a support on which her family depends, and thus they also bear connected risk. Her physical risks include all the risks associated with pregnancy, as well as with the higher-frequency multiple pregnancies associated with IVF. For example, despite the increased risks to their health, these subjects lack the insurance of long-term health care. One reason client parents stated for coming to India for surrogacy is that doctors are willing to transfer more embryos during implantation than in other countries such as the United States, the United Kingdom, or Israel. This increases the chances of success within a given cycle of IVF, but it also means that there is a higher frequency of multiple births and more frequent embryo reduction when multiple pregnancies occur. At Manushi, there is a policy of permitting only single or twin pregnancies for the protection of the mother and remaining fetus, but because compliance with the currently existing national guidelines is voluntary, policy is implemented idiosyncratically at the level of the individual clinic. The clinic will store frozen embryos for clients, but there is concern in India about the need for regulation of what happens to unwanted frozen embryos. A surrogate does not have a say regarding practices like embryo reduction and caesarian deliveries beyond her agreement with the clinic's general policy, and there is currently no state recognition of any legally-defensible connection between the surrogate and her direct family with the child to whom she gives birth. The children born to surrogates are also subject to risk, particularly as preliminary research suggests that people born through IVF, particularly with eggs from women over age 35, may be subject to increased risk of Down's Syndrome and other genetic diseases (Roberts 2011). The contracting or intended parents are also experimental subjects as they negotiate the legal meaning of parentage between national legal structures and ARTs.

The draws for commissioning parents to come to India for gestational surrogacy are many, and are interesting in how they reveal the interaction of culturally varied understandings of the meaning of gestation and childbirth with the choice and mobility offered by privatized and transnational structures of fertility therapies.[7] A recent study of medical tourism in India has identified that the two most common factors drawing travelers from wealthier countries to India are avoiding wait-times (in countries with socialized medicine), and seeking lower cost (in general) (Crooks et al. 2011). In additional to the availability of advanced technologies, highly trained physicians, and the low-cost of their services, there is also the seemingly easy availability of low-cost gestational carriers. I have argued elsewhere that there are false assumptions about the needs and necessary quality of life for Indian low-wage workers that underpin the naturalized "cheapness" of Indian labor in general, and the artificial production of the availability of inexpensive workers, including surrogates, in India (Vora 2009, 2015). This ethnography adds two other reasons that may be statistically less influential, but add to the picture of why commissioning parents travel to India for gestational surrogacy. The first is that fertility clinics in places where there is a profit motive in medicine tend to accelerate their procedures to the point where patients feel dehumanized and anonymous. In Indian clinics, which are by contrast service oriented in their transnational practices, despite being profit-motivated, patients seeking surrogates may find a more attentive, individualized and even caring interface and experience. Another is particular to diasporic/nonresident Indian patients and others who find accommodation in India for cultural, religious, or caste-based understandings of the meaning of the pregnant body and in its role in the transmission of culture and identity beyond the medical and property-based definition of parenthood. The discrepancy between the western medical narrative of genetic inheritance (Martin 2001) and conflicting cultural notions of what is inherited culturally through the womb has also been documented as a concern in ethnographies of gestational surrogacy in Israel (Teman 2010), Egypt (Inhorn 2003), and the United States (Thompson 2005).

While at first the expansion of ART clinics to accommodate transnational demand seems to expand general access to ARTs, a number of scholars have emphasized that access to such technologies continues to be highly limited by class and racial inequalities (Inhorn and Birenbaum-Carmeli 2008; Inhorn et al. 2008; Spar 2006). Also, as Marcia Inhorn has pointed out, infertility rates in the Third World itself are high, and there is a (largely unmet) demand for fertility services and technologies. In fact, fertility problems are a significant source of suffering and stigma in India (Inhorn and Bharadwaj 2007), and are part of a large-scale "global fertility problem" (Inhorn 2003, 1844). However, as she emphasizes, access to these technologies is limited only to those who are very wealthy in comparison to the majority of the population. She argues that improving access to primary care, more accessible than many ARTs, would have also have a significant effect in reducing infertility worldwide, because many infertility cases in her primary site of Egypt as well as other developing countries are caused by preventable conditions (Inhorn 2003, 1840). From her observation, we can add that increased emphasis at the level of the local clinic as well as at the national level as evidenced in draft ART legislation upon provision of fertility technologies to medical travelers from the Global North may redirect resources from the provision of care and the study, treatment, and prevention of the causes and symptoms of infertility among the same classes in India from which gestational surrogates originate.

The infertility rate in the demographic subset that encompasses the largest percentage of people in India, including the communities from which many of the women who become surrogates originate, is estimated to be 8–10%. This population holds low-paying jobs ranging from day labor to entry-level clerical work, service and small-manufacturing jobs, or are transitioning from small family farming to urban-based work because of being dispossessed from their land for reasons of environmental, legal, and agribusiness-related change. While the infertility rate of this population is high, only 2% of that 8–10% actually require ARTs for successful treatment; the vast majority of fertility problems are caused by poor health, substandard nutrition, poor maternity services, and high levels of infections (Inhorn and Bharadwaj 2007; Qadeer and John 2008). The vastly more lucrative business of providing fertility technologies to medical travelers from the Global North will likely undercut the provision of care and resources for studying, treating, and preventing the causes and symptoms of infertility among the same classes in India from which gestational surrogates originate.[8] Once a bill is passed by the Indian parliament as based on the current draft bill, governance of ART actors will continue to occur through highly problematic protections of market-based rights and market-compromised choice, identified even in the draft bill's preamble as oriented towards protecting the rights of commissioning parents as consumers first and foremost. As K. Sundar Rajan explains in his ethnographic work on "experimental values" and clinical trials in India, when governments must compete to attract commercial research organizations to their countries, they do this in part by offering laws attractive to them (2007), a situation which finds its parallel in national ART legislation that is oriented toward elite Indian and transnational consumers at the expense of surrogates and egg donors.

In the transnational ART clinic, we can observe medicine shifting from a technique of caring for the body to one of producing bodies as the instruments of service work as part of an experiment with engaging a transnational, technologically mediated market that depends on socially mediated arrangements with local, relatively low-resourced women surrogates. The body of the surrogate is rendered available as part of this experiment with gestation as a service. Transnational surrogacy in India points to some of the continuities and contradictions inherent in the evolution of relations between foreign economic demands, projects of the Indian elite and middle-class, and low-income rurally based Indians that have precedent in the colonial period. The relationship between foreign governance, Indian elites and the subaltern rural majority population of India tracked in the work of subaltern historiographies is evident in the nature of contact and socialities formed in the clinic, but with the added dimensions of the privatization and transnational commerce. To fully explore this topic is not within the confines of this chapter, but the clinic's context does suggest some important details. A relationship of power between the Indian middle and upper-middle classes, here the doctors running the clinic and elite Indian commissioning parents, and the rural, less educated, less connected, and much lower resourced women they hire to act as gestational surrogates represents in part a continuity with India's colonial past. At the same time, the transnational reach of clinic directors, and their ability to command technology and resources at a global level represents something unique though not unrelated to that historical relationship. The foreign commissioning parents also do not fit into this paradigm in a tidy way, as they are both consumers of the labor of surrogates, but also experimental subjects themselves, as they engage with both real and imagined relationships to the women who are acting as egg donors and gestational surrogates for them. Women participating as surrogates also add complexity to structural relations of dominance as they experiment with mutually supportive sisterly relationships in the hostels, as well as imagine the possible future relationships with commissioning parents that recast surrogacy as incommensurate with their surrogacy fee and leave commissioning parents beholden to them.

Conclusion

Reproductive technologies participate in the creation of new social contexts and forms of exchange between different groups in India and abroad, as well as to new meanings attached to them. In the transnational surrogacy clinic these groups can include upper-middle class clinicians, transnational and local patients who have the financial means to undergo fertility therapies, and lower-income local surrogates and egg donors. These exchanges, which include both market-based transactions as well as exchanges of an altruistic and/or gift nature, require management to control the kinds of social meanings that participants may attach to them. The clinic manages social meaning through narratives that narrowly define the relationship between technologies and the social meanings involved and created through surrogacy. Existing scholarship on transnational commercial surrogacy in India addresses concern within India and internationally that commercial surrogacy is a form of exploitation of the women working as surrogates (Pande 2009a, 2009b; Vora 2009). Scholarship has also raised urgent legal concerns about the lack of regulation of ARTs in general, and surrogacy practices in particular, in India (Smerdon 2008). These concerns are woven into the ways that medical staff attempt to control the social meaning attached to ARTs, and the ways that actors in the clinic experiment with different forms of sociality, trying out different roles and meanings within the surrogacy relationship. These experiments require novel approaches to understanding the social implications of ARTs.

Notes

1 Assisted reproductive technologies, which aid in conception and pregnancy, include practices such as hormonal inducement of ovulation, the harvesting of human ova for *in vitro* fertilization, and embryo transfer to the uterus along with hormones that aid in embryo implantation in the uterus and hence successful pregnancy.

2 I use the terms "commissioning parents" to refer to the individuals or couples who initiates the surrogacy process, in part to remain consistent with the language of draft ART legislation in India. The terms "intended parents" and "gestational surrogate" or "gestational carrier" are most often used in literature on ARTs and surrogacy in the Anglo-American academy. In the clinic, everyone referred to the women who carried pregnancies to term under contract to commissioning parents simply as "surrogates."

3 This term derives from Michel Foucault's lectures and publications where it is used to refer to techniques of government and citizen-subject that make a society governable in a given historical period.

4 All identifying information of people, places and institutions has been changed to protect identities while preserving a sense of the atmosphere or climate of informality in the clinic.

5 Although exclusively local donors were used at this clinic, one of the two commissioning couples I met that were using donated eggs was unaware of this fact. See Vora 2009.

6 In this case, a commissioning father from Japan was prevented from returning with an infant born to a surrogate in India because of legal complications concerning custody and citizenship between India and Japan. The intended parents divorced after entering a surrogacy arrangement through an Indian clinic, utilizing the intended father's sperm and donated eggs. The couple divorced before the delivery, and when the commissioning father attempted to return to Japan with the infant, a law in India preventing single men from adopting female children was invoked.

7 Aditya Bharadwaj has written extensively on the social contexts of ARTs in India, including discussion of the cultural, media, and political stakes involved

for different populations of Indians in engaging with reproductive technologies (2003, 2006).

8 Kaushik Sundar Rajan has written about a parallel situation in the context of clinical trials run by US-based pharmaceutical companies in India, where the context of risk includes the situation that participants who have positive outcomes have no guarantee of access to the drugs developed as a result of their trial (Rajan 2007, 78).

Works Cited

Arnold, David. (1988). "Touching the Body: Perspectives on the Indian Plague," in *Selected Subaltern Studies*, Ranajit Guha and Gayatri Chakravorty Spivak, eds. Oxford: Oxford University Press, pp. 391–426.

Arnold, David. (1993). *Colonizing the Body*. Berkeley: University of California Press.

The Assisted Reproductive Technologies (Regulation) Bill. (2010). "Indian Council of Medical Research," poster draft. www.icmr.nic.in/guide/ART&per;20REGULATION&per;20Draft&per;20Bill1.pdf.

Bharadwaj, A. (2003). "Why Adoption Is Not an Option in India: The Visibility of Infertility, the Secrecy of Donor Insemination, and Other Cultural Complexities," *Social Science and Medicine*, 56: 1867–1880.

Bharadwaj, A. (2006). "Sacred Modernity: Religion, Infertility, and Technoscientific Conception Around the Globe," *Culture, Medicine, and Psychiatry*, 30: 423–425.

Brouwer, Jan. (1999). "Modern and Indigenous Perceptions in Small Enterprises," *Economic and Political Weekly*, 34(48): 152–156.

Crooks, V.A., L. Turner, J. Snyder, R. Johnston and P. Kingsbury. (2011). "Promoting Medical Tourism to India: Messages, Images, and the Marketing of International Patient Travel," *Social Science & Medicine*, 72(5): 726–732.

Inhorn, M.C. (2003). "Global Infertility and the Globalization of New Reproductive Technologies: Illustrations from Egypt," *Social Science & Medicine*, 56: 1837–1851.

Inhorn, M.C. and A. Bharadwaj. (2007). "Reproductively Disabled Lives: Infertility, Stigma, and Suffering in Egypt and India," in *Disability in Local and Global Worlds*, B. Ingstad and S.R. Whyte, eds. Berkeley: University of California Press, pp. 78–109.

Inhorn, M.C. and D. Birenbaum-Carmeli. (2008). "Assisted Reproductive Technologies and Cultural Change," *Annual Review of Anthropology*, 37: 177–196.

Inhorn, Marcia C., R. Ceballo and R. Nachtigall. (2008). "Marginalized, Invisible, and Unwanted: American Minority Struggles with Infertility and Assisted Conception," in *Marginalised Reproduction: Ethnicity, Infertility and Assisted Conception*, Culley N. Hudson and F. Van Rooij, eds. London: Earthscan, pp. 181–198.

Martin, E. (2001). *The Woman in the Body: A Cultural Analysis of Reproduction*. Boston, MA: Beacon Press.

Pande, Amrita. (2009a). "It May Be Her Eggs But It Is My Blood: Surrogates and Everyday Forms of Kinship in India," *Qualitative Sociology*, 32(4): 379–397.

Pande, Amrita. (2009b). "Not an Angel, Not a Whore: Surrogates as Dirty Workers in India," *Indian Journal of Gender Studies*, 16(2): 141–173.

Prakash, Gyan. (1999). *Another Reason: Science and the Imagination of Modern India*. Princeton, NJ: Princeton University Press.

Qadeer, Imrana and Mary John (via Nivedita Menon). (2008). "Surrogacy Politics: Imrana Qadeer and Mary E. John," *Kafila*, December 25. http://kafila.org/2008/12/25/surrogacy-politics-imrana-qadeer-mary-e-john/. Accessed January 3, 2009.

Rapp, R. (1999). *Testing Women, Testing the Fetus: The Social Impact of Amniocentesis in America*. New York: Routledge.

Roberts, Michelle. (2011). "IVF Procedure 'May Increase Risk of Down Syndrome'," *BBC News: Health*, July 3. www.bbc.co.uk/news/health-13992232.

Saravanan, Sheela. (2010). "Maternal-Fetal Bonding in the Complex Setting of Transnational Commercial Surrogacy in India," presentation at the European Conference on Modern South Asian Studies, Bonn, Germany, July.

Smerdon, U. (2008). "Crossing Bodies, Crossing Borders: International Surrogacy Between the United States and India," *Cumberland Law Review*, 39(1): 15–85.

Spar, Deborah. (2006). *The Baby Business: How Money, Science, and Politics Drive the Commerce of Conception*. Cambridge, MA: Harvard Business Press.

Stabile, C. (1998). "Shooting the Mother: Fetal Photography and the Politics of Disappearance," in *The Visible Woman: Imaging Technologies, Gender, and Science*, P.A. Treichler, L. Cartwright and C. Penley, eds. New York: New York University Press.

Sundar Rajan, Kaushik. (2007). "Experimental Values: Indian Clinical Trials and Surplus Health," *New Left Review*, May–June: 67–88.

Tadiar, Neferti. (2009). *Things Fall Away: Philippine Historical Experience and the Makings of Globalization*. Durham, NC: Duke University Press.

Teman, E. (2010). *Birthing a Mother: The Surrogate and the Body*. Berkeley: University of California Press.

Thompson, C. (2005). *Making Parents: The Ontological Choreography of Reproductive Technologies*. Cambridge, MA: MIT Press.

Towghi, Fouzieyha and Kalindi Vora. (2014). "Bodies, Markets, and the Experimental in South Asia," *Ethnos: Journal of Anthropology*, 79(1): 1–18. DOI:10.1080/00141844.2013.810660.

Vora, Kalindi. (2009). "Indian Transnational Surrogacy and the Commodification of Vital Energy," *Subjectivity*, 28: 266–278.

Vora, Kalindi. (2011). "Medicine, Markets and the Pregnant Body: Indian Commercial Surrogacy and Reproductive Labor in a Transnational Frame," *Scholar & Feminist Online, Double Issue*, 9(1–2).

Vora, Kalindi. (2015). *Life Support: Vital Commodities Between India and the US*. Minneapolis, MA: University of Minnesota Press.

8

CITIZEN, SUBJECT, PROPERTY

Indian Surrogacy and the Global Fertility Market

International fertility travel engages structural inequalities that arise from histories of conquest, capture, and colonialism, and is entwined with the landscape of mobility, migration, and rights. To better understand these relationships and their effects on participants in transnational fertility markets, this chapter explores the ways that transnational surrogacy arrangements in India raise new issues around the legal and social construction of citizenship as a technology of mobility and the marking of rights-bearing subjects. Through a relational analysis of how differential citizenship has functioned to demarcate weak citizenship for low-earning subjects like women who become surrogates in India or women of color mothers in the United States, and by comparing historical instances where infants are regarded as property, aliens, or citizens in the United States and India, this chapter brings a new analytics to scholarship on the exposure of actors in surrogacy arrangements to risk in terms of long-term health and social consequences, precarity, and potential rightlessness.

After establishing the context of how the nation-based concept of citizenship has evolved, we reference Indian draft legislation intended to regulate ART practice together with recent case law that navigates the citizenship and mobility of infants who are born to Indian surrogates but are intended to have the foreign citizenship of their commissioning parents. We raise the question of how histories of labor and mobility structured into the current ordering of the postcolonial world influence the market for surrogacy and gametes. The notion of citizenship depends on legally enforced relations of labor and property, and, in the United States context, bridges the incommensurable yet not unrelated processes of human commodification involved in the 19th-century racial slavery and 21st-century transnational gestational surrogacy. By bringing recent research on surrogacy together with critical theoretical work on the construction of citizenship, we highlight the ways in which the practice of transnational commercial surrogacy both grows out of and reinforces structures of inequality produced and policed through the various apparatuses of the state.

DOI: 10.4324/9781003353362-8

We argue that when US commissioning parents contract Indian women as commercial gestational surrogates, they engage a structural history of the instrumentalization of the reproductive capacities of women who are marginalized by race, class, and the law for the benefit of subjects who are economically, legally, and socially more privileged. Putting analysis of the practice of US commissioning parents contracting commercial surrogacy in India into conversation with theories of citizenship and the nation-state, focusing in particular on US citizenship and its racial underpinnings, we suggest lines of inquiry for the ongoing scholarly examination of transnational surrogacy, but also suggest that discourses of citizenship might be strategically deployed in the policy arena in order to pursue a greater measure of rights and benefits for gestational mothers.

Background on Commercial Surrogacy in India

Commercial gestational surrogacy in India, born out of historical, social, and market inequities, is already a sociologically complex phenomenon increasing in volume and scope. Rapid growth in the surrogacy market is occurring without the resolution of legal inequalities and medical risks that are likely to affect surrogates, commissioning parents, and the children born from these arrangements. ART clinics in India currently are encouraged to adhere to national "guidelines," but are not actually bound by any enforceable legislation. There is also no mandatory reporting, so the full scope of practices can only be estimated. Research suggests that around 2000 babies were born to gestational surrogates in India in 2011. As many as 1000 are thought to have been commissioned by British client-parents, though figures involving British citizens may be underreported as commercial surrogacy is illegal in the United Kingdom (Knoch 2014). As of 2015, the number of clinics offering surrogacy services in India was roughly estimated to be between 600 and 700, and the Indian Council for Medical Research predicts that fertility travel to India will soon be a six billion dollar industry (Rudrappa 2012).

The first surrogacy clinics established in India catered primarily to North American, Israeli, Australian, and European clients, with additional clients from Taiwan, Japan, and Gulf nations. Newer clinics serve populations from Pakistan and Bangladesh where ART technology and practice is less available (Kashyap 2011), with a similarly motivated growth in clients from Tanzania, Nigeria, and Ethiopia (Deomampo 2013). Marcia Inhorn has argued that in nations where lack of preventative medicine is the primary cause of infertility, earlier intervention is more important than ART treatments for fertility issues in local populations (Inhorn 2003), and so ART isn't a demographic necessity for the local population. India is one such country, and despite the rapid development of fertility services this is not in the areas of necessity for local residents. Those with the resources to use

ARTs in nations that do not offer it often travel to other parts of the global south for ART services (Inhorn 2012). Thus, as Daisy Deomampo argues, there exists a complex, gendered, and racialized global geography of reproductive tourism (2013).

The long-term health impacts of gestational surrogacy are understudied, particularly in light of how rapidly the number of clinics offering this service is multiplying (Knoch 2014). Obstetrics research has shown that conception through IVF increases the risk of gestational hypertension, preeclampsia, placenta previa, hyperemesis gravidarum, venous thromboembolism, and cholestasis (Knoch 2014), and the low-resource context of women who become surrogates in India likely increases the chances of these complications, many of which can have long-term health consequences for women. Despite the fact that surrogates are at risk for serious adverse health effects, permanent injury, and death, ethnographic accounts make it clear that the surrogate is not seen as a patient in ART, but as a tool for commissioning parents who are the patients (Saravanan 2013; Vora 2009, 2012; SAMA 2012; Riggs and Due 2010). Surrogates are provided little information about the process of IVF, and though clinics may obtain formal consent through a signed form, in general surrogates are not treated as clinical subjects and therefore informed consent is not sought. Surrogacy contracts offer few protections for women in cases where long-term care becomes necessary. At that time, the Draft ART Bill (2012) required that commissioning parents pay for one year of medical insurance following the delivery of the infant, but the bill provides no rights, compensation, or care for the surrogate and/or her family in cases of longer-term illness or permanent injury. This lack of long-term protection means that the surrogacy arrangement has the potential to pose financial disaster for the surrogate's family, as well as medical disaster for the surrogate herself. Not only is the woman's regular income lost to the family if she is unable to return to her usual work due to a pregnancy-related injury; the family is also burdened with the financial costs of the woman's lifelong care. Adverse outcomes of pregnancy and delivery can include paralysis, blindness, need for repeated surgeries, and lifelong dependence upon medications to compensate for damaged organs. The single year of medical care proposed in the Draft ART Bill 2012 does not protect surrogates and their families from medical and financial devastation in such cases.

Most Indian surrogates and their spouses work in the informal economic sector, and therefore receive low wages with unstable employment and few if any benefits, despite sometimes unsafe working conditions that can endanger their health (SAMA 2012, 58). Ethnographic research shows that surrogates and their families

> often do without many necessities that commissioning parents would not do without, including basic health insurance, medical

> privacy, reliable electricity, clean and reliable water, a permanent home/residence, the ability to seek and find another job when one is lost, access to a variety of foods or the ability to grow them (requiring land and water), and so on.
>
> (Vora 2012, 687)

Many are in situations of "acute financial desperation" (Pande 2014, 49). This type of financial desperation on the part of potential surrogates, along with India's technological, medical, and economic infrastructure, makes it possible for commissioning parents from the global North to avail themselves of surrogacy services in India much more cheaply than they could in their home countries.

The ability of United States and other transnational clients to utilize Indian women as gestational surrogates at a significantly lower cost than they would pay to contract with women in their home countries must be understood within the context of the global historical and economic structures that have produced both the economic desperation of potential surrogates in India and the relative wealth of potential clients in the global North. The fact that large populations in India go without adequate food, clean water, medical care, education, and other necessities is a historical and structural co-constituent of the superabundance that middle-class US families are able to take for granted. The violently enforced designation of land and human populations in the historically colonized and currently neo-colonized world as sites of extraction for the enrichment (financial and otherwise) of both public and private interests in the First World maintains the material conditions of lack, want, and scarcity under which Third World women are impelled to enter surrogacy contracts with relatively wealthy US and other transnational clients, for a financial sum that represents a mere fraction of what those clients might pay for a surrogate in their own country. The lower fee for Indian surrogates does not reflect a geopolitical-economic order in which Indian families can access the same life-giving resources as US families for less money; it reflects a geopolitical-economic order in which Indian families are materially positioned to live with a lower level of these life-giving resources.

The nature of transnational surrogacy in India is further obscured by less-than-accurate assumptions about who the participants are—i.e., whose labor is making the surrogacy process possible. While only the clients, the medical staff and surrogacy brokers, and the surrogate herself are named in the contract, the entire arrangement is also underpinned by the labor of the surrogate's family. Surrogacy clinics often require surrogates to live away from their families, in clinic-run hostels, throughout their pregnancies (Vora 2011). The family—notably the surrogate's own children—thus, bear the affective burden of making the surrogacy possible via this prolonged familial separation. Additionally, the labor normally performed by the woman within her household must presumably be taken on by other family members during her absence. The mandate that surrogates reside in hostels also speaks to the artificially low cost of transnational surrogacy in India: when clinics require surrogates to live in hostels so they can be assured of getting nutritional foods, clean water, and medical services during pregnancy, the obvious reason for this requirement is that the surrogates' usual family lives do not include such benefits. Rather than paying enough for a surrogate's family to eat a variety of healthy foods, drink consistently safe water, and access professional medical care, the clinic can simply require the surrogate to leave her family and stay in a hostel. This requirement ensures that the surrogate has sufficient nutritional benefits and health protections during the pregnancy, in order to promote the optimum health and development of the clients' future child. If the surrogate's own children become sick from contaminated water or from a lack of variety in their diet, the surrogacy brokers and commissioning parents need not bear any financial cost or even be affectively troubled with the knowledge of such details. The bulk of the surrogacy fee is generally paid upon successful delivery of the infant to the commissioning parents, but given the uncertainty of this outcome, a woman could undergo six or seven months of pregnancy (with all of its accompanying dangers and discomforts), separation from her family, and absence from her normal paid employment, only to have a miscarriage which (in addition to potentially endangering her own life) means that the whole process has resulted in a net financial loss for her family.

The exponential growth of the transnational surrogacy market in India speaks to the satisfaction of international clients, who see in India an amenable and affordable location for the outsourcing of reproductive labor. At the same time, what is experienced by clients as the low cost of surrogacy arrangements in India is actually produced through the enforcement of a de facto lower standard of living and more limited conception of rights for the subaltern Indian classes from which surrogates are drawn. And while the fees promised upon successful completion of the pregnancy are many times what the woman would make at her regular work, the exposure of the surrogate's body and family to long-term risk and potential rightlessness gets elided in the limited understanding of surrogacy as a 9-month labor contract.

Race and Reproduction in the Construction of Citizenship and Property

The conditions of possibility for transnational surrogacy in India, in addition to involving new developments in biotechnology, arise from very old structures of imperialism and race. In this regard, the different types of human commodification involved in 19th-century racial slavery and 21st-century Indian gestational surrogacy, while clearly distinct and incommensurable, are not unrelated. Thinking about economies of slavery, particularly in terms of US history, both provides historical context for the current positionality of middle-class US clients (as having the means to outsource the bodily labor of biological reproduction) and helps to set up an analytic lens for an examination of the relationships between citizenship, noncitizenship, and the commodification of reproduction.

During the 17th and 18th centuries, evolving structures of race and empire gave rise to an international economic order founded upon the circulation of captive humans as commodities. The commoditized human body played a foundational role in the political and economic development of the US settler state (Takaki 2000). Even before separation from England, white settlers in what would eventually become "the United States" had developed a profitable economy grounded in the labor of enslaved Blacks and Indians. By the 19th century, the profitability of the enslaved Black body for the white owner (or potential owner) was understood to be divisible into a number of constituent components: slaves too old or sick to work could be sold to medical colleges or to individual scientists for experimentation and dissection, and the reproductive capacity of the enslaved Black woman was regarded as possessing a financial value separate from and in addition to her capacity for field labor or domestic work (Morgan 2004). The enslaved Black woman had the potential to give birth to children who would inherit their mother's slave status; hence, to purchase a female slave was to invest in a self-multiplying commodity (Ibid.). To pay a higher price for an enslaved female regarded as a "breeder," or for a visibly pregnant enslaved woman, was to speculate in futurity, to make an investment toward the predicted financial value to be had from lives-yet-to-exist. After the formal banning of the transatlantic slave trade in 1808, the still rapidly expanding domestic slave trade relied entirely upon the reproductive capacities of enslaved Black women (Harrison 2009). Legal studies scholar Dorothy Roberts was one of the first Black feminist scholars to draw attention to how the market in reproductive labor was prefigured by the dependence on the US economy under slavery on the reproductive capacities of women who were enslaved (Roberts 1996). Kalindi Vora traces the continuities in contemporary outsourcing back to British colonial labor allocation. When slavery was abolished in the British Empire in 1807, indentured Indian workers were brought in to supplement slave labor (2015). Vora then traces the ways that Indian laborers have continued to be figure as best fit for service work and easily replaceable in the global outsourcing market. In that theoretical framing, surrogacy can be seen as part of an international division of reproductive labor that includes India's role in artificially cheapened service economies that were part of the growth of outsourcing. This is on a continuum with Winddance-Twine (2011) and Weinbaum (2019) who have centered in their engaging of Indian commercial surrogacy in the context of the commodification of Black women's reproductivity under slavery.

When the 21st-century US clients use their position within the global market and the gendered international division of labor in order to utilize Indian women's wombs for the purpose of reproducing their own genetic material, these clients are not engaging commodified human reproductivity as a new phenomenon; rather, their very ability to take advantage of transnational surrogacy arrangement is historically rooted in generations of commodified human reproductivity. This process also recapitulates racialized constructions of citizenship and noncitizenship, as we will now discuss.

Racialized Constructions of Citizenship and Noncitizenship

Gestational surrogates in India lack full protection as Indian citizens as a result of their low-earning status and as contracted workers in a transnational agreement. "Citizenship," notes Lynn Fujiwara (2008) "is a multilayered construct at constant play on the local, national, and international political terrain."[1] The notion of citizenship serves as an instrument for sorting and classifying bodies and subjects. The hegemonic status of the concept of citizenship naturalizes the ability of the nation-state to prescribe and enforce notions of who belongs where, of which bodies are allowed to move into and out of which geopolitical spaces, and when, and under what circumstances. Within the US context, citizenship, like property, has always been constructed through the technology of race. In this regard, Cheryl Harris' well-known analysis of "whiteness as property" provides a generative model for the analysis of US citizenship (1993)

Harris outlines the ways in which the legal construction of property in the United States settler state has been co-constituted with the social construction of race. The development of the US economy, and of the US state itself, has been predicated upon a racialized system of property, a system based on "the valorization of whiteness as treasured property in a society structured on racial caste." The 19th-century Market Revolution, the formative historical "moment" for the US settler state as a political and economic entity, hinged upon a particular set of articulations between racial identity and property: Indigenous people were displaced and killed in order to free up land which could then become the basis of white property; whites had the potential to own this property, while blacks were enslaved and therefore could not own property because they were legally figured as property. Later in the 19th century, the construction of "Asian" as a racial identity became linked to an ambivalent set of relationships to property: Asians could sometimes hold property, but could also have their property—including citizenship-as-property—revoked on the basis of their nonwhite status (Ngai 2004). Applying Marx's labor theory of value, we can note that the value of whiteness as property has always been produced through the labor of people excluded from the category of whiteness.

The formal abolition of slavery did not divest whiteness of its property value. Property acquired through whiteness was not re-distributed in the post-Civil War era, nor was there a radical legal disruption of the settled expectation that whiteness should confer special status (Harris 1993). The expectations attached to the notion of whiteness were not dismissed or refused post-bellum. Because the law continued to recognize and protect "expectations grounded in white privilege (albeit not explicitly in all instances)," these settled expectations remained "tantamount to property that could not permissibly be intruded upon without consent."

The reasoning behind Harris' analysis of whiteness as property also applies to US citizenship. The property value of legal status as a US citizen or resident, like the property value of whiteness, is dependent upon exclusivity, upon "the absolute right to exclude" (282). The material benefits of US citizenship, like the material benefits of whiteness, depend upon the structural relationship between a designated privileged group (US citizens) and its various nonprivileged others (people of the Third World, particularly in geopolitical areas that have a distinct neocolonial relationship with the United States). We can also note that the social constructions of whiteness and US citizenship are articulated together in the sense that federal law and policy around who is and is not eligible to become (and remain) a US citizen have historically been inseparable from notions of race and whiteness (Lopez 1996). Of course, the differential nature of US citizenship means that not all US citizens are able to derive the same level of enjoyment of their citizenship-as-property. The same can be said about whiteness as property: as race is inflected by other social constructions such as gender, sexual identity, and socioeconomic class, the fact that all whites possess whiteness-as-property does not mean that all whites can leverage this property to the same degree. Whiteness and US citizenship are thus similar to other property-forms in that they do not possess the same use-value for all who hold them, though they do consistently possess value-in-the-abstract and hence do constitute property for all who possess them.

Applying a Marxist analysis to an understanding of US citizenship as property leads to a number of provocative questions and insights, many of which have implications for the issue of transnational surrogacy. Posing again the question raised by the labor theory of value, we ask: Who performs the labor that becomes congealed as value in the form of US citizenship? During the 19th-century Market Revolution, the alienated labor of enslaved people became congealed not only in the form of white property and whiteness-as-property, but also in the form of US citizenship-as-property.[2] US citizenship today, in addition to containing the alienated and congealed labor of generations of enslaved people, also increases its value by absorbing the alienated and congealed labor of subjects who produce for the US nation-state but are not permitted to enter or legally inhabit the geopolitical space for which the fruits of their labor are destined. Indian gestational surrogates fall within the category of Third World workers who produce value for the US state and who labor toward the increase of US citizenship-as-property, but who are not allowed to legally inhabit the US state and hence do not have access to this type of valued property themselves.

Indian gestational surrogates produce commodities for the United States, for artificially depressed compensation, that reflect a global economic order featuring unequal exchange between the global North and South. On this very basic level, gestational surrogates are like Third World garment workers, or like the undocumented immigrants who labor in fields producing American food, or in cleanrooms producing American digital equipment. But gestational surrogacy centrally involves affective and biological labor, involving the commodification of unquantifiable processes extracted from Indian workers and re-invested in US families, US communities, and US society-at-large (Vora 2015).

Transnational Indian surrogacy arrangements offer commissioning parents bearing US citizenship an opportunity to utilize services by low-earning Indian citizens with limited mobility and of relatively weak citizenship in India, and to convey their citizenship status with its historical accretion of value to a child born by a woman without legal access to that status. Lisa Lowe notes that, "In the last century and a half, the American citizen has been defined over against the Asian immigrant, legally, economically, and culturally (IA, 4)." Transnational surrogacy arrangement preserve the privilege/property of commissioning parents residing in their citizenship, which depends on the exclusion of undesirable subjects, "reproducing the capitalist relations of production as racialized gendered relations and are therefore symptomatic and determining of the relations of production themselves" in a way that complements the history of immigration law in the United States (Lowe 22).

Inside the State, Outside the Protections of Citizenship

As Fujiwara notes, recent theories of citizenship highlight the politics of closure whereby some citizens are in fact excluded from full participation, resulting in a de-facto structure of differential citizenship. We need only recall the extensive history of state-sanctioned violence against Black citizens simply attempting to exercise the most basic citizen-activity of voting, in order to realize that differential citizenship: (1) is nothing new in the United States, and (2) is a co-constituent of the social construction of race. Evelynn Nakano Glenn (2004) highlights the distinction between formal citizenship and substantive citizenship. While formal citizenship "is that embodied in law and policy," substantive citizenship entails "the actual ability to exercise rights of citizenship" (53). Black Americans were granted birthright citizenship with the passage of the Fourteenth Amendment in 1868, thereby formally gaining such legal rights as "the right to vote"; however, their legal status as citizens often did not, in practice, lead to the protection of such formally-articulated rights. Furthermore, Glenn suggests that substantive citizenship goes beyond the protection of legal and political citizenship rights. Citing T.H. Marshall's classic concept of "social citizenship," Glenn points out that "the right to a modicum of economic security, education, and other resources" is obviously "necessary to realize one's civil and political rights."

Fujiwara suggests that scholars have tended to focus either on the study of legal citizenship or on issues of social citizenship, leading to the sense that "a tendency has emerged to examine citizenship at two disconnected levels." In reality, these different valences of citizenship are inextricably imbricated—and are caught up together in a vicious circle: Just as factors such as access to education and "a modicum of economic security" are necessary to an individual's or community's realization of civil and political rights, citizenship as legal status is necessary to the individual's or community's effective pursuit of things like meaningful education and fair employment.

Over the past few decades, developments in technology and finance have become incorporated into, and thereby modified, the structuring of differential citizenship. Aihwa Ong (1999) uses the term flexible citizenship to denote the ways in which both nation-states and individual citizens (as individuals per se and as members of families and communities) bend the citizenship binary and take advantage of this flexibility in order to pursue a range of goals—from national prestige and the growth of national economies, to individual and familial financial profits, to social mobility and a sense of economic security. Citizenship is "flexibilized" when the law and public policy position particular regions, populations, activities, and individual bodies as simultaneously within and outside of the nation-state. Ong points to the suspension of national labor laws and other protections in "export processing zones" (also known as "special economic zones," "free trade zones," etc.); workers entering these zones lose many of the rights and protections they would otherwise possess as citizens of the nation-state. They are "inside" the state, but "outside" the protections normally afforded to citizens of the state.[3]

Flexible citizenship is not only a nation-state strategy; it is also refers to the ways in which individuals and kinship groups utilize their own citizenship in "flexible" ways, and take advantage of the "flexibility" of the nation-state system in order to promote their interests. "In this sense," Ong writes, "'flexible citizenship' also denotes the localizing strategies of subjects who, through a variety of familial and economic practices, seek to evade, deflect, and take advantage of political and economic conditions in different parts of the world." Such strategies include collecting multiple passports, sending offspring to study in particular nation-states in order to establish business and social connections in those areas, etc. State regimes "are constantly adjusting" to fluctuating trends in the global circulation of both money and bodies (Ong 1999).

Flexible and differential citizenship comes into play on both sides of the transnational surrogacy equation in India. Potential surrogates, though they hold formal citizenship in the Indian state, do not have social citizenship in T.H. Marshall's sense; their families do not have access to things like education or "a modicum of economic security"; indeed, it is these things that they are attempting to access through participation in the surrogacy process. Furthermore, the ART clinic—indeed, the surrogate's body itself—becomes like an "export processing zone," in which the rights of the subaltern Indian citizen (i.e., the surrogate) are suspended in the interest of cheap, efficient production for the transnational client. The woman who becomes pregnant through ART under a surrogacy contract, though she remains inside the geographic borders of the Indian state, is outside of the protections normally afforded to Indian citizens: since the ART clinic is not legally bound to follow the national "guidelines" regarding surrogacy, the woman is not protected by the nation-state and is instead essentially "governed" by the clinic, an institution which—as stated earlier—regards her less as a patient than as a means of production. At the same time, the clients in transnational Indian surrogacy arrangements, while benefitting from the surrogate's lack of social citizenship in her home country and the flexibilization of her citizenship status once she enters the surrogacy clinic, simultaneously benefit from their own "strong" US citizenship to exercise forms of cross-border mobility and rule-bending. Deomampo's ethnographic work shows how US clients argue with US and Indian officials and insist that rules and procedures be changed in order to accommodate their preferred timelines for leaving India with their surrogate-produced infants. Flexible citizenship thus facilitates the transnational surrogacy process: for the surrogate, the rights of citizenship are flexibilized; for the clients, the rules of citizenship (and borders) are flexibilized. The infant produced by the surrogate's body, labor, and vitality, ceases to be a commodity as soon as it is delivered to its intended recipients, the commissioning parents. Thereafter, the infant is no longer a commodity, but a self-authenticating subject of rights: a citizen. Under the current US legal system, the infant produced through surrogate gestational labor inherits, not the non-citizen status of the mother who gives birth to it, but the citizen status of the commissioning parents whose gametes have been used to produce the embryo implanted into the surrogate.

Under US law, birthright citizenship is conferred according to two principles: *jus soli*, or the "right of the soil," and *jus sanguinis*, the "right of the blood." Prior to 1868, birthright citizenship was the exclusive provenance of whites—a long-standing fact that was reconfirmed with the 1857 Dred Scott case, in which the Supreme Court declared that persons of African descent could not be regarded as citizens of the United States. With the 1868 passage of the Fourteenth Amendment, birthright citizenship was conferred upon the descendants of slaves, along with all other "persons born or naturalized in the United States, and subject to the jurisdiction thereof."

The phrase "subject to the jurisdiction thereof" was used to exclude Native Americans born within reservations or tribes, although these individuals clearly were subject to US jurisdiction in practice. Birthright citizenship was granted to Native Americans as a group in 1924, with the passage of the "Indian Citizenship Act."

As compared with *jus soli*, the legal adjudication of *jus sanguinis* is currently much less clear-cut. The mythical notion of American "blood" suggests that anyone who has such "blood" should naturally have US citizenship. While the foreign-born offspring of US citizens are generally granted US citizenship on the principle of *jus sanguinis*, there are many cases in which such offspring are in fact not given US citizenship. The granting of US citizenship to a child born outside the United States is contingent upon a number of factors, including whether or not the parents are married, whether or not both parents are US citizens, whether or not the father acknowledges the child, and whether or not the US citizen parent (if only one parent is a US citizen) has resided within the United States for a total of at least 5 years, at least 2 years of which residence must have been after the US citizen parent's 14th birthday.

Not being eligible for *jus soli*, the children produced by Indian surrogates on behalf of US commissioning parents are considered US citizens on the basis of *jus sanguinis*. Of course, the actual "blood" that produces the child is not "American," nor does the subject-body that produces this blood have the opportunity to gain the status of US citizen (Pande 2009). Nevertheless, the child is a US citizen on the basis of *jus sanguinis*. The mother whose blood has produced the child, by contrast, remains a subaltern citizen of the Indian state.

The Latin term *jus sanguinis* becomes confusing and contradictory in the context of granting birthright citizenship to an infant generated and birthed through the blood of an Indian surrogate mother 9 months after implantation of an embryo produced in an Indian lab using gametes from a US couple. Under these conditions, a different term is perhaps needed in order to more accurately reflect the basis upon which the infant is considered a US citizen. *Jus gametas*? Vora also notes that in cases where the female of the commissioning pair cannot produce a viable egg, an egg from an Indian donor may be used (Vora 2013, 98). In such special cases of *jus gametas*, when the child is generated through the blood and bloodshed of an Indian birth mother 9 months after implantation of an embryo produced in an Indian lab from an Indian donor's egg and a US citizen's sperm, is the sperm-father required to prove that he has met the 5-year US residency requirement, with at least two of those years of residency having taken place after his fourteenth birthday? Or is the infant granted US citizenship on the basis of *jus spermae*?

It is interesting to note that the connection between kinship and citizenship implied by the principle of *jus sanguinis* has traditionally functioned in multiple directions: not only can foreign-born offspring of US-citizen parents gain US citizenship through this principle, but (naturalized or *jus soli* birthright) US citizens over the age of 21 can petition for permanent US residency status for their foreign-born parents and siblings, who can then become naturalized US citizens on this basis. Indian surrogate mothers who give birth to US citizen children are unique in this regard: they produce US citizens, but are granted no corresponding ability to become US citizens.

Conclusion

By producing value for US society while remaining forcibly outside of that society themselves, Indian surrogates valorize US citizenship. In this regard, they are structurally similar to Third World sweatshop workers, and to various (historical and contemporary) noncitizen laboring populations within the United States. But Indian surrogates are unique in that the extraction of their vital energy not only enhances the property value of US *citizenship*, but also biologically reproduces the *citizenry* itself. In this sense, transnational gestational surrogacy in fact represents an entirely new phenomenon. While the labor of producing the property-value of US citizenship has always been "outsourced," so to speak, the rise of transnational surrogacy represents the outsourcing of the cellular-biological reproduction of the US citizenry. In these ways, we have argued that different valences of citizenship are inextricably imbricated in transnational India surrogacy, and need to be considered in assessing access to rights and entitlements by and for subjects of surrogacy arrangements.

Notes

1 Lynn Fujiwara, *Mothers Without Citizenship: Asian Immigrant Families and the Consequences of Welfare Reform*, p. 24.

2 Though Marx, by his own admission, specifically does *not* structure his critique of political economy around an analysis of chattel slavery, the use of Marxist concepts and language to discuss chattel slavery in America is not without precedent. Also, despite the fact that he did not engage with chattel slavery in a sustained manner, Marx did acknowledge that "the veiled slavery of wage workers in Europe needed, for its pedestal, slavery pure and simple in the new world." The following passages from *Capital Volume I* are also relevant here:

> Liverpool waxed fat on the slave trade. This was its method of primitive accumulation. And, even to the present day, Liverpool "respectability" is the Pindar of the slave-trade which . . . 'has coincided with that spirit of bold adventure which has characterised the trade of Liverpool and rapidly carried it to its present state of property; has occasioned vast employment for shipping and sailors, and greatly augmented the demand for the manufactures of the country.

[The U.S. cotton industry provided] a stimulus to the transformation of the earlier, more or less patriarchal slavery, into a system of commercial exploitation. In fact, the veiled slavery of the wage-workers in Europe needed, for its pedestal, slavery pure and simple in the new world.

The discovery of gold and silver in America, the extirpation, enslavement and entombment in mines of the aboriginal population, the beginning of the conquest and looting of the East Indies, the turning of Africa into a warren for the commercial hunting of blackskins, signalised the rosy dawn of the era of capitalist production.

3 Ong gives the example of export processing zones in Indonesia: "Large export-oriented industrial zones are located in Sumatra and Java; they depend on cheap labor to manufacture furniture, watches, clothing, shoes, toys, and plastic goods. Millions of young women have left their rice fields to work for less than a living wage in factories operated by Koreans that subcontract for brand-name companies such as Nike, Reebok, and The Gap. But besides making Indonesia part of the global production system, these industrial estates are institutional contexts of limited citizenship: workers are rarely protected by the state, are in fact frequently harassed by the military, and are left to adjust as well as they can to the exigencies of the market" (Ong 1999, 222–223).

Works Cited

Cooper, Melinda and Catherine Waldby. (2014). *Clinical Labor: Tissue Donors and Research Subjects in the Global Bioeconomy*. Durham, NC: Duke University Press.

Deomampo, Daisy. (2013). "Gendered Geographies of Reproductive Tourism," *Gender & Society*, 27(4): 514–527.

Deomampo, Daisy. (2014). "Defining Parents, Making Citizens: Nationality and Citizenship in Transnational Surrogacy," *Medical Anthropology: Cross-cultural Studies in Health and Illness*, 34.

Fujiwara, Lynn. (2008). *Mothers Without Citizenship: Asian Immigrant Families and the Consequences of Welfare Reform*. Minneapolis, MA: University of Minnesota Press, 24.

Glenn, Evelynn Nakano. (2004). *Unequal Freedom: How Race and Gender Shaped American Citizenship and Labor*. Cambridge and London: Harvard University Press.

Harris, Cheryl I. (1993). "Whiteness as Property," *Harvard Law Review*, 106(8).

Harrison, Renee K. (2009). *Enslaved Women and the Art of Resistance in Antebellum America*. New York: Palgrave Macmillan.

Indian Council of Medical Research, Ministry of Health and Family Welfare, Govt. of India, New Delhi. 2012.

Inhorn, Marcia C. (2003). "Global Infertility and the Globalization of New Reproductive Technologies: Illustrations from Egypt," *Social Science & Medicine*, 56: 1837–1851.

Inhorn, Marcia C. (2012). "Reproductive Exile in Global Dubai: South Asian Stories," *Cultural Politics*, 8: 283–306.

Kashyap, Pooja. (2011). "Test Tube Babies No Real Option in Patna," *Times of India*, October 20.

Knoch, Jonathan K. (2014). "Health Concerns and Ethical Considerations Regarding International Surrogacy," *International Journal of Gynecology & Obstetrics*,

April 27. www.sciencedirect.com/science/article/pii/S0020729214002276. Accessed May 15, 2014.

Lopez, Ian Haney. (1996). *White by Law: The Legal Construction of Race*. New York: New York University Press.

Morgan, Jennifer. (2004). *Laboring Women: Reproduction and Gender in New World Slavery*. Philadelphia, PA: University of Pennsylvania Press.

Ngai, Mai. (2004). *Impossible Subjects: Illegal Aliens and the Making of Modern America*. Princeton, NJ: Princeton University Press.

Ong, Aihwa. (1999). *Flexible Citizenship: The Cultural Logics of Transnationality*. Durham, NC: Duke University Press.

Pande, Amrita. (2009). "It May Be Her Eggs but It Is My Blood: Surrogates and Everyday Forms of Kinship in India," *Qualitative Sociology*, 32(4): 379–397.

Pande, Amrita. (2014). *Wombs in Labor: Transnational Commercial Surrogacy in India*. New York: Columbia University Press.

Riggs, Damien W. and Clemence Due. (2010). "Gay Men, Race Privilege and Surrogacy in India," *Outskirts: Feminisms Along the Edge*, 22.

Roberts, Dorothy. (1996). "Race and the New Reproduction," *Hastings Law Journal*, 47(4): 935–949.

Rudrappa, Sharmila. (2012). "Working India's Reproduction Assembly Line: Surrogacy and Reproductive Rights?," *Western Humanities Review*, 66(3): 77–96.

SAMA: Resource Group for Women's Health. (2012). *Birthing a Market: A Study on Commercial Surrogacy*. New Delhi: SAMA. www.samawomenshealth.org/downloads/Birthing%20A%20Market.pdf.

Saravanan, Sheela. (2013). "An Ethnomethodological Approach to Examine Exploitation in the Context of Capacity, Trust and Experience of Commercial Surrogacy in India," *Philosophy, Ethics, and Humanities in Medicine*, 8(10): 1–12.

Takaki, R. (2000). *Iron Cages: Race and Culture in 19th-Century America*. New York: Oxford University Press.

Vora, Kalindi. (2009). "Indian Transnational Surrogacy and the Commodification of Vital Energy," *Subjectivities*, 28: 266–278.

Vora, Kalindi. (2012). "Limits of Labor," *South Atlantic Quarterly*, 201(111): 681–700.

Vora, Kalindi. (2013). "Potential, Risk and Return in Transnational Indian Gestational Surrogacy," *Current Anthropology*, 54(suppl. 7): S97–S105.

Vora, Kalindi. (2014). "Experimental Socialities and Gestational Surrogacy in the Indian ART Clinic," *Ethnos: Journal of Anthropology*, 79(1): 63–83.

Vora, Kalindi. (2015). *Life Support: Biocapital and the New History of Outsourced Labor*. Minneapolis, MA: University of Minnesota Press.

Weinbaum, Alys Eve. (2019). *The Afterlife of Reproductive Slavery: Biocapitalism and Black Feminism's Philosophy of History*. Durham and London: Duke University Press.

Winddance-Twine, Francis. (2011). *Outsourcing the Womb: Race, Class and Gestational Surrogacy in a Global Market*. New York and London: Routledge.

9

CONCLUSION

After the Housewife: Surrogacy, Labor, and Human Reproduction

Human reproduction in the form of pregnancy, childbirth, breastfeeding, and nurturing of infants and children has been at the core of Marxist feminist understandings of reproductive labor. When this labor is overtly commercialized, as in the case of surrogacy, it brings together biological processes of gestational and social processes of nurture and parenting into market relationships. Just as feminist scholars have had to work to theorize how domestic labor, sex work, and service are economically and socially productive activities, researchers are now extending and building upon those theories to encompass practices like commercial surrogacy as hired human reproduction, and in general the biological processes of bodies (i.e., clinical trial subjects) and tissues (novel cells in the lab that come from an individually important body) as sites that generate economic value.

Commercial gestational surrogacy is a practice in which someone enters a paid contract to gestate an embryo and deliver an infant for one or more commissioning (also called "intended") parents. Embryos are created by in vitro fertilization, a lab-based process in which ova from an intended mother or donor are fertilized with sperm from an intended father or donor. The resulting embryo (or embryos) is then transferred to the uterus of the gestational carrier, which has been prepared by hormones to allow the embryo to attach, and thereby start pregnancy and gestation.

In late 2015, just before transnational surrogacy arrangements were banned in India, there were as many as 3000 operating clinics.[1] At the Manushi clinic in northwestern India, where I conducted ethnographic research on transnational surrogacy arrangements between 2008 and 2015, surrogates were highly encouraged to move into residence hostels after the first trimester of pregnancy. Here, they would eat a regulated diet, receive regular preventative medical exams in line with the Euro-American standards of prenatal care, and participate in sanctioned activities which the clinic described as preserving them from manual and other paid work, as well as household work for their own families. These conditions were described by current surrogates as very different from pregnancies with their own

DOI: 10.4324/9781003353362-9

children, which were almost exclusively overseen by local midwives outside the clinic and the practice of allopathic medicine.

The surrogate is a complicated subject of labor. First, there is the social location of surrogacy as mothering labor and the cultural economic weight of the household/family economic unit that comes with that location. Second, gestation and childbirth are imbricated with the body and subject of the surrogate in a way that makes it difficult to distinguish between what is labor and what is not. Finally, because women becoming surrogates in India are at a disadvantage in terms of financial resources, political influence, mobility and access to knowledge, the idea that surrogacy contracts are freely entered with informed consent is also complicated.[2] Moreover, the women I spoke to who were pregnant as surrogates offered their own theories of what surrogacy was: for instance, many described the value and meaning of surrogacy as different from a job, as apart from categories of kinship new or old, and as apart from clinic and market discourses. There was instead an emphasis on a feeling that carrying a child for a couple that could not otherwise have a child was something so extraordinary that it was almost a divine act; this aspect of the arrangement was more important than money as a motivation.

> Discourse about the divine aspects of surrogacy point to simultaneous and competing logics for the social meaning and value of gestational surrogacy. These meanings cannot be easily organized or communicated through the genetic definition of a biological parent, though it is a condition of possibility for commercial surrogacy, or even through the economic logic of the value of the labor of surrogacy as underpaid and technologically mediated "women's work" in the global economy.[3]

My argument, then, is that commercial surrogacy involves both biological and affective labor (e.g., self-care and surveillance in addition to gestation), but also produces value through more than just labor.[4] Like most forms of gendered labor, these biological and affective processes are difficult to separate from the body and person of the woman acting as a surrogate. This makes the work of surrogacy a form of labor that engages histories of race and colonialism and at the same time, in the reproduction of the human that supports social reproduction, pertinent to the arguments of materialist feminists for the need to classify and compensate reproductive labor.

Transnational Surrogacy Contracts in India

The context in which women enter surrogacy contracts as their best employment option, which includes privatization of land and other resources, resulting in the loss of family farms, and a subsequent shift to urban employment, is one where entering surrogacy is like entering the industrialized workforce. Yet, because these conditions engage the history of colonialism, which instrumentalized consent, freedom and choice, alienation, and sexual and reproductive relations that do not register as "labor," it is easy to overlook them.[5] The history of India's rule as a colony to be exploited for labor and resources left infrastructure that continues to affect the hyper-availability of racialized and gendered bodies.[6] The emergence of women in working and lower middle-class India as gestational surrogates fits into a pattern where advances in biotechnology make the bodies and body parts of workers more sellable and mobile than their labor, what Lawrence Cohen calls "bioavailability."[7] The structural adjustment policies to liberalize India's economy in the early 1990s contributed to the conditions under which women cannot find sufficient work other than by finding some way to make their value travel to meet capital when labor migration is not financially possible, here through transnational surrogacy. In fact, Kamala Kempadoo argues that neoliberal reforms imposed by the World Bank and IMF upon these formerly colonized nations have effectively been a process of recolonization of female, reproductive work.[8] While all biological life represents a site of speculation and potential biological production and accumulation, the legacies of imperialism continue to affect the hyper-availability of racialized and gendered bodies. In the case of transnational gestational surrogacy contracts in India, which were in practice between 2004 and 2016 when the practice was officially banned, the colonial prehistory of contemporary globalization and outsourcing of labor and laboring populations influences how we can understand the very nature of the work being performed.[9]

The biological and affective nature of women's participation as surrogates under paid contract challenges the analytical frameworks most often used to quantify or even identify an activity as labor. As scholars studying the bioeconomy have argued, this challenge to the labor categories of political theory characterizes a number of emerging biological markets.[10] However, contrary to the newness of the technologies that make gestational surrogacy contracts possible, the difficulty in accounting for embodied and therefore gendered labors of care, affect and the body is not new. In fact, both materialist feminist analysis of housework and black feminist analysis of women's reproduction and bodies under chattel slavery have raised problems with the labor theory of value and the privileging of the subject of labor. For example, Leopoldina Fortunati has argued that reproductive labor has a dual function in capitalism—work occurring in the domestic or otherwise nonpublic realm that produces service, whether bodily, physical or emotional, represents itself and the person performing it as nonvalue, yet it simultaneously channels the value it actually does produce into the capitalist system through the visibly productive workers who consume it.[11]

Maria Mies explains that the modern marriage contract sets up a model of unpaid labor in the private sphere, the home, that is then extended through globalization to encompass the formerly colonized world's labor economies.[12] We can add casualized labor, including many forms of crowdsourced digital labor and sweatshop work, as extending from this model of unpaid and under-paid labor in the gendered private sphere. The former colonial metropole, in the position of patriarch, commands the gendered labor of globalized service economies in the position of "wife"—sweatshop garment work, customer service call center work, long-distance tutoring and distance education, or crowdsourced microtask work like that managed by platforms such as Amazon mechanical turk. These forms of labor have little in common except that they are deemed to be uncreative or reproductive, and therefore while they are performed by people of any gender, the work itself is feminized, a process that Mies called "housewifization."

After the Housewife

Contracted surrogacy involves a spectrum of intimate and bodily actions that are still being theorized and catalogued as labor. As the paid work of pregnancy, gestation, and childbirth, surrogacy falls into a category of bodily work in the private sphere that is not only devalued in Fortunati's terms, but becomes difficult to regulate, and given the limits on other choices and informed consent, walks a line between free and coerced participation. In the context of transnational commercial surrogacy contracts, the intended parent then becomes the commissioning parent, a type of profit-based patient. Doctors, formerly agents of pastoral care, become paid service providers who manage the technical, medical, and social supervision of the process being commissioned. The clinic provides a portal for the transition of surrogates into the global service economy and ironically, their transition into an industrialized labor force.

Women of color feminists have critiqued the racialized nature of domesticity and free labor, whether or not it is performed in the home, pointing out that capitalism has grown not just because of so-called productive and reproductive labor, but also through the exhaustion of life past the possibility of its reproduction.[13] For example, the reproductive labor and bodies of women under slavery weren't comparable to unpaid housewives, as enslaved women were legally considered property, rather than a subject who could exchange labor for a wage. Children born to women under slavery remained slaves, and therefore the property of slave owners. The domination of women under slavery meant that the first issue of concern wasn't the lack of the wage for their work; it was the fact that they were property, rather than subjects who could sell their labor.

Other women of color feminists in the United States, including Evelyn Nakano Glenn and Grace Chang among others, have pointed out that immigrant and low-resourced women have always done their own household labor, plus additional under-paid wage labor in the households of wealthier, often white, families.[14] Angela Y. Davis also argues that historically, the reproductive work of the household in Black families has not been socially valued in the United States. For example, in 1971, Davis described the domestic or reproductive work of women under slavery in the United States, which was performed not in the family household, but for men and children who were not necessarily a family group under conditions of complete domination. She goes on to theorize this domestic space as the main space of resistance, because this reproductive labor was the only work not fully claimed by the slave owner, and while reproducing the lives of the enslaved, also created the conditions for resistance.[15] In the early 1980s, Davis critiqued the "Wages for Housework" campaign by arguing that Black women and other women of color had been performing paid housework for decades, in other words making housework a public responsibility, and that this had not improved the valuing of that labor, which was still low-waged work. Supplementing Fortunati's argument about middle class white women's labor in the household, Jennifer Morgan explains that Black women's bodies were as essential to the success of chattel slavery as their labor in the antebellum US south.[16]

Like domestic workers in the home who create the opportunity for middle-class women to work outside the home, outsourced service work is supposed to supply lower-valued, often feminized tasks so that other workers can be freed to do more highly valued, masculine tasks. First performed by women, then by hired women of color and female immigrant workers, and finally sent to overseas workers, these tasks do not lose the association of being feminized and therefore unskilled, resulting in low compensation and social valuing. New technologies, like the biotechnologies discussed earlier, have historically marked what kinds of labor are considered replaceable and reproducible, and those that are productive and therefore highly valued. Long-distance telecommunications allowed for the outsourcing of voice-based customer service, and the Internet extended this to text- and visual-based labor.

Surrogates, like the figure of the housewife in the Wages for Housework campaign, but also other workers isolated to labor in the private sphere including domestic workers and intellectual pieceworkers doing crowd-sourced work, among increasing numbers of others, have inherited the feminization, and therefore devaluation of the home as a workplace. They are also positioned in a global division of labor that has mapped itself onto the decolonizing world to feminize developing labor markets. At the same time that commercial surrogacy upholds Davis's point that the "housewife" is limited as a bourgeois figure that represents only the tip of the iceberg of women's labor and experience, surrogacy illustrates the enclosure and expropriation of women's bodies discussed by Silvia Federici.[17] More than the class-specific, race delimited and advanced capitalist location of the housewife, Federici's observation of the enclosure of women's bodies to harness and control reproductive capacity explains why commercial surrogacy is continuous with the logic of capitalist accumulation via women's bodies and reproductivity.

Surrogacy as a Site of Resistance?

Bringing together materialist feminist, women of color critique, and contemporary work on reproduction presents an urgent need to decolonize reproduction and to imagine domestic labor as a site of resistance. In the case of surrogacy, this should include empowering the models for sharing of resources advocated for by surrogates who see their work as above and beyond what can be represented by a labor contract, which imposes a regime of property and privacy where many surrogates expect ongoing social relation and reciprocity.[18] In my ethnographic study of surrogacy, women who were currently engaged in surrogacy contracts talked about the value and meaning of surrogacy in two ways. On the one hand, there was the feeling that such bodily work, so closely associated with adultery as carrying the child of a man not your husband), was dangerously stigmatizing.[19] On the other hand, there was an emphasis on a feeling that carrying someone else's child was extraordinary, almost divine. While the need for income was the impetus to become a surrogate, this extraordinary aspect of surrogacy was much more heavily weighted, and in fact, inspired a common-sense expectation for ongoing social relations and social support of their own families by the commissioning parents. In this sense, women refused the alienation of the commercialization of their surrogacy through the contract, insisting on its meaningfulness as social reproductive activity even though it is outside the area on the household proper. These women undertaking surrogacy thus describe their understanding of the risks and future potential of their work in terms that acknowledge, but also exceed the clinic's discourse of surrogacy as simply the paid service of gestation and rented use of an otherwise unused uterus. Their "unreasonable" expectation of a sense of indebtedness on the part of commissioning parents could be seen as an attempt to "potentialize" relationships formed through the clinic and to stabilize one of the competing meanings of surrogacy as exceeding what is represented by the contract.

Notes

1 It is difficult to get comprehensive statistics for the nature and outcome of births associated with ART clinics in India right now because there is no required reporting (SAMA Resource Group for Women and Health 2010).

2 See Kalindi Vora. (2012). "Limits of Labour: Accounting for Affect and the Biological in Transnational Surrogacy and Service Work," *The South Atlantic Quarterly*, 111(4): 681–700; Kalindi Vora (2015b). *Life Support: Biocapital and*

the New History of Outsourced Labour (Minneapolis, MA: University of Minnesota Press).
3 Kalindi Vora. (2013). "Potential, Risk and Return in Transnational Indian Gestational Surrogacy," *Current Anthropology*, 54(Suppl. 7): S97–S106.
4 See Kalindi Vora. (2015a). "Re-Imagining Reproduction: Unsettling Metaphors in the History of Imperial Science and Commercial Surrogacy in India," *Somatechnics,* 5(1): 88–103; Kalindi Vora. (2014). "Experimental Sociality and Gestational Surrogacy in the Indian ART Clinic," *Ethnos: Journal of Anthropology*, 79(1): 1–18; Kalindi Vora, "Limits of Labour."
5 See Vora, "Limits of Labour"; *Life Support*; "Re-Imagining Reproduction."
6 Vora, "Re-Imagining Reproduction."
7 Lawrence Cohen. (2004). "Operability: Surgery at the Margins of the State," in Anthropology in the Margins of the State, Veena Das and Deborah Poole, eds. (Santa Fe, NM: School of American Research Press), 79–106.
8 Kamala Kempadoo. (1999). "Continuities and Change: Five Centuries of Prostitution in the Caribbean," in Sun, Sex and Gold: Tourism and Sex Work in the Caribbean, Kamala Kempadoo, ed. (New York and Oxford: Rowman & Littlefield).
9 Vora, *Life Support.*
10 See Catherine Waldby and Melinda Cooper. (2008). "The Biopolitics of Reproduction," *Australian Feminist Studies*, 23(55): 57–73; Catherine Waldby and Melinda Cooper. (2010). "From Reproductive Work to Regenerative Labour: The Female Body and the Stem Cell Industries," *Feminist Theory,* 11(1): 3–22; Melinda Cooper and Catherine Waldby. (2014). *Clinical Labour: Tissue Donors and Research Subjects in the Global Bioeconomy* (Durham, NC: Duke University Press); Kaushik Sunder Rajan. (2006). *Biocapital: The Constitution of Postgenomic Life* (Durham, NC: Duke University Press).
11 Leopoldina Fortunati. (1989). The Arcane of Reproduction: Housework, Prostitution, Labour and Capital, trans. Hilary Creek, ed. Jim Fleming (New York: Autonomedia).
12 Maria Mies. (1986). *Patriarchy and Accumulation on a World Scale* (London: Third World Books).
13 Angela Y. Davis. (1998). "Reflections on the Black Woman's Role in the Community of Slaves," in *The Angela Y. Davis Reader*, Joy James, ed. (London: Blackwell), 111–129; Grace Hong. (2012). "Existential Surplus: Women of Colour, Feminism and the New Crisis of Capitalism," *GLQ: A Journal of Lesbian and Gay Studies,* 18; 87–106; Jennifer Morgan. (2004). *Labouring Women: Reproduction and Gender in New World Slavery* (Philadelphia, PA: University of Pennsylvania Press).
14 Evelyn Nakano Glenn. (1992). "From Servitude to Service: Historical Continuities in the Racial Division of Paid Reproductive Labour," SIGNS: Journal of Women and Culture in Society, 18; 1–43; Grace Chang. (2004). Disposable Domestics: Immigrant Women Workers in the Global Economy (Cambridge, MA: South End Press).
15 Davis, 'Reflections on the Black Woman's Role'.
16 In *Labouring Women*, Morgan writes, "The obscene logic of racial slavery defined reproduction as work, and the work of the colonies—creating wealth out of the wilderness—relied on the appropriation of enslaved women's children by colonial slave owners . . . The effort of reproducing the labour force occurred alongside that of cultivating crops" (145). Jennifer Morgan. (2004). *Laboring Women: Reproduction and Gender in New World Slavery* (Philadelphia, PA: University of Pennsylvania Press).

17 Silvia Federici. (2004). Caliban and the Witch: Women, the Body and Primitive Accumulation (Oakland, CA: Autonomedia).
18 See Vora, "Experimental Sociality"; *Life Support*; "Re-Imagining Reproduction."
19 See also Amrita Pande (2009). "Not an Angel, Not a Whore: Surrogates as Dirty Workers in India," *Indian Journal of Gender Studies*, DOI:10.1177/097152150901600201.

Works Cited

Cooper, Melinda and Catherine Waldby. (2014). *Clinical Labor: Tissue Donors and Research Subjects in the Global Bioeconomy*. Durham, NC: Duke University Press.

Chang, Grace. (2000). *Disposable Domestics: Immigrant Women Workers in the Global Economy*. Cambridge, MA: South End Press.

Cohen, Lawrence. (2004). "Operability: Surgery at the Margins of the State," in *Anthropology in the Margins of the State*, Veena Das and Deborah Poole, eds. Santa Fe, NM: School of American Research Press, pp. 79–106.

Davis, Angela Y. (1983). "The Approaching Obsolescence of Housework: A Working-Class Perspective," in *Women, Race & Class*. New York: Vintage Press.

Davis, Angela Y. (1998). "Reflections on the Black Woman's Role in the Community of Slaves," in *The Angela Y. Davis Reader*. Malden, MA: Blackwell Publishers, pp. 111–129 (reprint of 1971 original).

Federici, Sylvia. (2004). *Caliban and the Witch: Women, the Body and Primitive Accumulation*. New York: Autonomedia.

Fortunati, Leopoldina. (1989). *The Arcane of Reproduction: Housework, Prostitution, Labor and Capital*, Jim Fleming, ed. and Hilary Creek, trans. New York: Autonomedia.

Glenn, Evelyn Nakano. (1992). "From Servitude to Service: Historical Continuities in the Racial Division of Paid Reproductive Labor," *SIGNS: Journal of Women and Culture in Society*, 18: 1–43.

Hong, Grace. (2012). "Existential Surplus: Women of Color, Feminism and the New Crisis of Capitalism," *GLQ: A Journal of Lesbian and Gay Studies*, 18: 87–106.

Jakobsen, Janet. (2012). "Perverse Justice," *GLQ: A Journal of Lesbian and Gay Studies*, 18(1): 25.

Kempadoo, Kamala. (1999). "Continuities and Change: Five Centuries of Prostitution in the Caribbean," in *Sun, Sex and Gold: Tourism and Sex Work in the Caribbean*, edited by Kamala Kempadoo. New York and Oxford: Rowman & Littlefield.

Mies, Maria. (1986). *Patriarchy and Accumulation on a World Scale: Women in the International Division of Labor*. London: Third World Books; Atlantic Highlands, NJ: Zed Books.

Morgan, Jennifer. (2004). *Laboring Women: Reproduction and Gender in New World Slavery*. Philadelphia, PA: University of Pennsylvania Press.

Pande, Amrita. (2009). "Not an Angel, Not a Whore: Surrogates as Dirty Workers in India," *Indian Journal of Gender Studies*, 16(2): 141–173. https://doi.org/10.1177/097152150901600201

SAMA Resource Group for Women and Health. (2010). *Unraveling the Fertility Industry: Challenges and Strategies for Movement Building*. New Delhi: International

Consultation on Commercial, Economic, and Ethical Aspects of Assisted Reproductive Technologies. www.samawomenshealth.org/downloads/Final%20Consultation%20Report.pdf.
Sunder Rajan, Kaushi. (2006). *Biocapital: The Constitution of Postgenomic Life*. Durham, NC: Duke University Press.
Vora, Kalindi. (2012). "Limits of Labour: Accounting for Affect and the Biological in Transnational Surrogacy and Service Work," *The South Atlantic Quarterly*, 111(4): 681–700.
Vora, Kalindi. (2013). "Potential, Risk and Return in Transnational Indian Gestational Surrogacy," *Current Anthropology*, 54(Suppl. 7): S97–S106.
Vora, Kalindi. (2014). "Experimental Sociality and Gestational Surrogacy in the Indian ART Clinic," *Ethnos: Journal of Anthropology*, 79(1): 1–18.
Vora, Kalindi. (2015a). "Re-Imagining Reproduction: Unsettling Metaphors in the History of Imperial Science and Commercial Surrogacy in India," *Somatechnics*, 5(1): 88–103.
Vora, Kalindi. (2015b). *Life Support: Biocapital and the New History of Outsourced Labour*. Minneapolis, MA: University of Minnesota Press.
Waldby, Catherine and Melinda Cooper. (2008). "The Biopolitics of Reproduction," *Australian Feminist Studies*, 23(55): 57–73.
Waldby, Catherine and Melinda Cooper. (2010). "From Reproductive Work to Regenerative Labour: The Female Body and the Stem Cell Industries," *Feminist Theory*, 11(1): 3–22.

INDEX

For Product Safety Concerns and Information please contact our EU representative GPSR@taylorandfrancis.com Taylor & Francis Verlag GmbH, Kaufingerstraße 24, 80331 München, Germany